End of Life

Nursing Solutions for Death with Dignity

Lynn Keegan, RN, PhD, AHN-BC, FAAN, is director of Holistic Nursing Consultants in Port Angeles, Washington. She is one of the founders of the holistic health focus in nursing and a well-known leader in holistic nursing. She has authored or coauthored 18 books as well as scores of professional journal publications and chapters in textbooks. Some of her books include five editions of the coauthored, three-time *American Journal of Nursing* award-winning Book of the Year textbook, *Holistic Nursing: A Handbook for Practice* (5th ed., 2009); *Healing Nutrition* (1st and 2nd ed.); *Healing with Complementary and Alternative Therapies; Healing Waters: The Miraculous Health Benefits of Earth's Most Essential Resource; Profiles of Nurse Healers;* and *The Nurse as Healer,* among others. In addition, she has delivered scores of presentations and keynote addresses in numerous countries throughout the world.

Dr. Keegan was elected as a Fellow of the American Academy of Nursing and is board certified as an Advanced Holistic Nurse by the American Holistic Nurses Association. She is past president of the American Holistic Nurses Association and is on the board of many organizations and journals. She has served on the faculty of several prominent universities, working at multiple levels, from teaching associate degree programs all the way through coordinating graduate nursing programs. In 1991 she received the Distinguished Alumnus Award from Cornell University–New York Hospital School of Nursing.

Carole Ann Drick, PhD, RN, TNS, TNSCP, is director of Conscious Awareness, Inc., in Austintown, Ohio. She is one of the early organizers and supporters of the holistic health focus in nursing as well as a known leader in holistic nursing. She has authored or coauthored two books and numerous professional publications. Most recently she authored *Mother Stories: Through Our Mothers' Death and Dying* (2007), 16 true stories of women and the gifts they received while remaining with their mothers during the death and dying process. She, along with Lynn Keegan and another coauthor, wrote *American Holistic Nursing Association: Implementing Visions of Health and Healing* (2008), published by the American Holistic Nurses Association. She has four consciousness CDs plus more in production. She is an active national and international speaker.

Dr. Drick studied with the International Fellowship of Introspection, receiving Teacher of Natural Science certification plus a Teacher of Natural Science Certifying Practitioner Certification, of which there are only two currently in the world. She served the American Holistic Nurses Association as chair of the Education Approver Committee in the early 1980s and resumed the position in 2006. In 2010 she became the practice coordinator for the association. She has been on the graduate faculty of two large universities and has developed and implemented a new baccalaureate nursing program based on holistic principles and adult teaching and learning strategies. She served on the editorial board of the *Journal of Holistic Nursing* for many years.

End of Life

Nursing Solutions for Death with Dignity

LYNN KEEGAN, RN, PhD, AHN-BC, FAAN
CAROLE ANN DRICK, PhD, RN, TNS, TNSCP

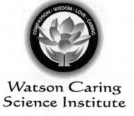

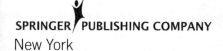
SPRINGER PUBLISHING COMPANY
New York

Watson Caring
Science Institute

Springer Publishing Company, LLC
11 West 42nd Street
New York, NY 10036
www.springerpub.com

Acquisitions Editor: Margaret Zuccarini
Production Editor: Gayle Lee
Cover Design: Joseph DePinho
Project Manager: Laura Stewart
Composition: Apex CoVantage

ISBN: 978-0-8261-0759-6
E-book ISBN: 978-0-8261-0760-2

10 11 12 13 14/ 5 4 3 2 1

Library of Congress Cataloging-in-Publication Data

Keegan, Lynn.
  End of life : nursing solutions for death with dignity / Lynn Keegan, Carole Ann Drick.
    p. ; cm.
  Includes bibliographical references.
  ISBN 978-0-8261-0759-6 (alk. paper) — ISBN 978-0-8261-0760-2 (e-book) 1. Hospice nurses.
2. Terminal care. I. Drick, Carole Ann. II. Title.
  [DNLM: 1. Hospice Care. 2. Nursing Care. 3. Advance Care Planning. 4. Attitude to Death. 5. Palliative Care. WY 152.3]
  RT87.T45K44   2011
  616'.029—dc22   2010032173

The author and the publisher of this Work have made every effort to use sources believed to be reliable to provide information that is accurate and compatible with the standards generally accepted at the time of publication. Because medical science is continually advancing, our knowledge base continues to expand. Therefore, as new information becomes available, changes in procedures become necessary. We recommend that the reader always consult current research and specific institutional policies before performing any clinical procedure. The author and publisher shall not be liable for any special, consequential, or exemplary damages resulting, in whole or in part, from the readers' use of, or reliance on, the information contained in this book. The publisher has no responsibility for the persistence or accuracy of URLs for external or third-party Internet Web sites referred to in this publication and does not guarantee that any content on such Web sites is, or will remain, accurate or appropriate.

Special discounts on bulk quantities of our books are available to corporations, professional associations, pharmaceutical companies, health care organizations, and other qualifying groups.

If you are interested in a custom book, including chapters from more than one of our titles, we can provide that service as well.

For details, please contact:

Special Sales Department, Springer Publishing Company, LLC
11 West 42nd Street, 15th Floor, New York, NY 10036-8002
Phone: 877-687-7476 or 212-431-4370; Fax: 212-941-7842
Email: sales@springerpub.com

Printed in the United States of America by Hamilton Printing

Contents

Foreword

Jean Watson, PhD, RN, AHN-BC, FAAN

This work by Drs. Keegan and Drick, long-time leaders in holistic nursing, holds new visions of hope for nursing and human caring approaches and invites us back to our heart as the source for new and old visions, reflecting inner spaces, and considerations of places appropriate for dying and death. It is in the authors' vision of a *Golden Room* where they open to us methods and models through which values and actions reflect the depths of humanity and our evolved views for human kind in the completion of the great sacred cycle of living and dying. It is in this text and the vision of the *Golden Room as a nursing solution for death with dignity,* where we once again experience wisdom, compassion, caring, and love to the fullest and deepest. It is here where we reconnect with death notions and authentic expressions of tenderness, loving kindness, peace, beauty, grace, safety, pain-free honorable release, and safe space for the final passage in the cycle of life. The *Golden Room,* as a transcendent, transpersonal metaphor, reminds us of the inner recesses of our soul and the timeless journey we each seek in making our way back to mystery and the unknown—the soul's passage *home.* All humans need to respond to this call from beyond and awaken to how we wish to have dying and death honored and received. This work offers us a hopeful new reality for nursing and humankind to consider.

Both contemporary and futuristic, this work stands as a special gift to nursing and healing practitioners, humanity itself, as well as to all clinical systems, which need to hear and respond to this call for options supportive of this sacred trajectory from living to dying. It offers the possibility of ultimate healing and wholeness for individuals and society alike.

This work is a magnificent exemplar of the evolving work in Caring Science. It is a unique honor to have this work included

Dr. Jean Watson is Distinguished Professor of Nursing and Endowed Chair in Caring Science at the College of Nursing, University of Colorado, Denver. She is founder of the Watson Caring Science Institute in Boulder, Colorado.

in the Watson Caring Science Institute–Springer Publication Caring Science Library Series. It is a joy and privilege to endorse this critical work. The comprehensive dimensions and focus in this publication will pass the test of time. It serves as a guide, bringing us into a new era of human consciousness for the relevance of the precious, sacred circle of living and dying.

When one falls into the depth of Caring Science scholarship and holistic practices, one is drawn into the ethic, the philosophical grounding, of an emerging world-view—a cosmology that unites, connects, explains, and helps to order our very living–dying human reality, our chaotic world. It offers a new order of human evolution that embraces the paradox, the chaos, and the disorder. It offer's a new lens to understand, to comprehend, to personalize, to professionalize, and to give scientific and wisdom insights into creative emergence for what might be called the *ontological development* or *ontological design caring–healing* programs, projects, and purposive transformative practices that inform and authenticate human existence, human caring, and healing across the sacred life–death timeline of all of humanity.

Foreword

Barbara Dossey, PhD, RN, AHN-BC, FAAN

Every once in a long while a short, succinct book comes along that awakens our senses and motivates us to action. *End of Life: Nursing Solutions for Death with Dignity* is one such book. It cuts right to the chase to offer a new, innovative change for an old, outmoded rite of passage. In this instance the passage is literal, the passage from physical life to physical death.

Most contemporary deaths occur in the hospital or nursing home and may or may not be accompanied by the presence of loved ones. Often the experience involves varying levels of pain and suffering. Pain is the physical and/or emotional discomfort of symptoms. Suffering is the story around pain that may be physical, mental, emotional, social, and/or spiritual.

Death is not something people in contemporary American society prepare for, and certainly do not like to talk about. Death, for most, occurs in a hidden environment, secreted from children, and after it is over, is mourned as sorrowful.

Two well-known nurse scholars offer an innovative, inspired solution to the plight of the dying. Drs. Keegan and Drick have created a model of end-of-life care that occurs in a new, enlivened setting. *The Golden Room* is a metaphor for a specially built center that offers personalized, loving care at the end of life. What a novel idea. The ritual of birth is well developed with ceremony, special delivery units, and family-centered care. On the other hand, death is still hushed and for the most part isolated from celebration.

When my mother died, we held a unique and family-centered rite of passage for her. She departed this life in the midst of her loving family who were at her bedside all during the week-long passage to the other side. We held her, stroked her, and offered her all the comforts we knew she enjoyed. My dear mother's

Dr. Barbara Dossey is codirector of the Nightingale Initiative for Global Health in Ottawa, Ontario, Canada; and Arlington, Virginia. She also is director, Holistic Nursing Consultants in Santa Fe, New Mexico.

passage ritual was unusual, but to this day all of us who experienced this blessed event knew it was the right thing to do and the right setting to be in.

End of Life: Nursing Solutions for Death with Dignity offers rationales for both developing special dying locales and changing how we view and value death and the dying process. Once the reader understands the need for such places, the authors offer a model for a place for death with dignity: *Golden Room* centers. Read on, as I have, and become convinced that we have before us a new plan to aid and comfort each of us, who will inevitably die.

Preface

End of Life: Nursing Solutions for Death with Dignity considers how we, as professional nurses, can strive to advance death and dying to the next level in our evolution of compassionate end-of-life practices. The work focuses on describing the development of a place for dying that allows for a peaceful, profound experience that honors and respects human dignity and elevates the human family.

Unusual is the death that occurs in a gentle and loving environment. For most dying individuals and their families, this final physical life event is confounded by the acute care setting replete with all its manifest technology and incessant clinical care.

End of Life: Nursing Solutions for Death with Dignity presents a more conscious and humane way to experience death and dying. At present most anticipated deaths occur in hospital intensive care units, nursing homes, and/or hospice situations. The term *anticipated death* means not traumatic or accidental. Anticipated deaths represent the majority of people who succumb to old age or terminal illnesses such as cancer, heart disease, or pneumonia. *End of Life: Nursing Solutions for Death with Dignity* offers the opportunity to value and dignify this last most significant human event—physical death. Actual places called the *Golden Room* or *Golden Room* centers are proposed to accommodate dying persons and their loved ones as they make the transition from physical life. In essence, this book details a return to the *sacredness* of death and dying through access to a *place* for the physical *transition*.

Now is the time; here is the place—in the final hours of life, which we all will face—for a final decision for goodness, compassion, peace, dignity, and release. The plea is heard and answered in *End of Life: Nursing Solutions for Death with Dignity*.

Acknowledgments

Our book flows out of our culture's need for expanded attention to the dying process: where, how, and with whom one makes one's final transition. This book acknowledges all those who have already parted this earth and who, through their passing, have, one by one, increased our consciousness of why we need to continue to develop the process of a respectful and sacred death with dignity.

Our precious guide, Margaret Zuccarini, executive acquisitions editor, manifested herself to us at precisely the right time and the right place in this book's evolution. Her invitation to work with Springer Publishing to bring this work to fruition was heart centered and very welcome. Her insight and guidance helped us move this book from an idea into concrete reality. To Margaret, we are so grateful. We also appreciate the work of Elizabeth Stump, Margaret's assistant, who helped with the graphs. Gayle Lee, production editor at Springer, took the completed manuscript and navigated us through the refinement process. We thank you, Gayle. Special thanks to Laura Stewart, project manager, who skillfully edited and helped fix all the little details to make the book so readable. The team at Springer Publishing is an efficient, forward-thinking group of professionals who are exciting to work with. We thank all of them.

Special thanks to Jean Watson and her team at the Watson Caring Science Institute. They have had the foresight and courage to lead nurses worldwide into a conscious, caring practice. Nurses who have been touched by Jean and her caritas message alter their practice to include an enlightened approach to all who suffer and seek healing.

To the many thousands of holistic nurses, hospice nurses, and palliative care nurses who have been the leaders in the end-of-life, death-with-dignity movement, we thank you. These compassionate-care individuals and groups have paved the way for generations of nurses to come. Each member of our collective civilization will eventually face death, and through the work of these myriad numbers of on-the-job nurses, the final passing of each individual will be made better. To all of these dedicated nurses we offer a special thank you.

End of Life

Nursing Solutions for Death with Dignity

Part I

Foundations

1 *Why People Die*

As a cause of death the United States has no classification of "old age" even though dying from old age is very common.

—Unknown

*U*NCLE JOHN'S STORY   *By the time John was 93 years old he was alone and living in an Alzheimer's facility. His only remaining kin were two nephews. The older nephew, Tim, was designated John's power of attorney since John was now unable to care for himself. Prior to this point, John signed a living will wanting a peaceful death. Within a year John became incontinent, combative, and disagreeable with the staff. Increasing his medications was ineffective. Choosing not to deal with the problem, the facility owners told the nephews to find John a new home.*

John was transferred. Within a few weeks, his fight with another resident resulted in facial bruises and cuts for both men. The administrator recommended a psychologist, and his medications were altered again. After another fistfight the following week, a new problem began. At age 94 John began to manifest a variant of the Alzheimer's symptoms: sexual exposure and advances to demented Alzheimer's women. John was sent by ambulance to the local emergency room, where he was labeled a sexual predator and unsafe to house.

Tim worked with the on-call psychiatrist, mental health workers, and hospital staff to have John admitted to the local community hospital and then transferred to a geriatric psychiatry unit at a regional medical center for evaluation and medication adjustment.

John was discharged and placed in another facility. Within days John struck a female caregiver, breaking her nose. With more medications John finally settled down. His gait changed from a walk to a shuffle, and his eyes became glazed and disinterested.

On John's 95th birthday he began rectal bleeding. He could go to the hospital for tests or he could remain where he was and probably bleed to death. Not understanding the consequences, Tim authorized having John admitted to the acute care setting.

After four days of multiple tests, blood transfusions, and a colonoscopy, the diagnosis was diverticulitis/diverticulosis. The treatment would be antibiotics, followed by discharge back to the Alzheimer's facility. The next morning John complained of leg pain after falling out of bed and was returned to the hospital for an X-ray, which was normal. A magnetic resonance imaging (MRI) scan was scheduled as John still complained of leg pain. The tentative diagnosis was a possible fractured hip needing a surgical repair procedure. Another X-ray was ordered to check for any metal devices, such as an artificial hip. The X-ray and the MRI followed the next day. Both tests were negative; John returned to the nursing home.

John was given morphine for comfort, but he was not swallowing and therefore could not eat. The doctors speculated that he might have had a stroke. A feeding tube was proposed by the physician; the nephews decided against this life-prolonging method.

John continued his downhill course. Tim wavered, thinking the feeding tube might be a good idea. Tim did not understand the medical system or the physiological effects on an elderly frail body, including incontinence and, most commonly, buttocks decubiti, that eliminate most hope for a comfortable dying process.

On Sunday Tim suggested to the doctor that maybe they should try a feeding tube. Following a long pause, the doctor asked Tim, "What is your goal?" These four simple words are perhaps the most powerful ones to say when helping families reach decisions. There would be no recovery to quality life. Tim relented and accepted the inevitable.

Sunday night, John was transferred to hospice service only to find the IV was failing. The nephews conferred about a subclavian line and decided against this next life-prolonging option. On Monday John was having Cheyne–Stokes respiration, and his lungs were filling with fluid. On Tuesday evening, after 48 hours of pain and misery that incurred incredible hospital costs, John finally passed away.

The brothers and their wives were filled with guilt. They asked themselves and each other whether they might have made a better decision. John died alone in his hospital room. None of the distant family members slept well for many days following John's passing.

REFLECTIONS ON ISSUES OF CONCERN

1. Does diagnosis and treatment of conditions in a terminally ill, elderly, demented person contribute to the person's quality of life? The life of the family?
2. Who pays for the enormous, end-stage, acute care costs of Uncle John? Who should pay: the family or the government?
3. Who helps the family during the transition period?
4. In a time and place of teaching hospitals, should families be expected to pay for diagnosis and treatment when the primary benefit is the education and practicum experience of student and resident health care providers?
5. Life extension since the advent of antibiotics means more people are experiencing chronic debilitating diseases and painful deaths. What ethically can the health care system do to decrease the complications and pain for people who die from these diseases?
6. Cardiovascular disease accounts for about one-third of deaths. How does the concept of cardiovascular disease differ from the "natural causes" of death 50 years ago? Which way would you prefer to die?
7. Intentional injuries (suicides, violence, war, etc.) account for approximately 2.8% of deaths; traffic accidents cause 2.0%; suicides 1.5%. What can we do about preventable deaths such as these?
8. Cancer is expected to exceed cardiovascular disease as a cause of death in 2010. What statement is this making about the effectiveness of treatment? What causes of cancer are not being addressed? Are there cures used in other parts of the world that would benefit Americans?

The human soul is infinite, and yet when it comes to the actual physical process of death and dying we as health care professionals have a lot to remember. Often times during the dying process the focus is on care for and attention to bodily functions. Because of this directed attention and busyness we sometimes forget we are more than just a physical body. During the dying cycle it can be helpful for nurses and caregivers to pause and to recall that we and our dying loved ones are more than physical beings. We are also mind and spirit. Periodic pauses and conscious refocusing help us to remember and embrace the other dimensions of self. It is skilled and conscious caregivers who can best refocus simple physical care into directed intention and develop a greater wholeness to better assist the departing and his or her family as the dying person slips away. How did we ever allow advanced technology to take the place of the old and timeless values of compassionate end-of-life care? This book reviews the past and envisions the future possibilities of how the physical, emotional, and spiritual death process can become beautiful, peaceful, and dignified.

We invite you to explore why and when people die as the opening prelude to addressing the quality of end-of-life care and what we can do to enhance that experience, personally and professionally. Health care professionals know that many issues come up during the end-of-life period. Not only is there recognition of the physical end to life but also a need for emotional and spiritual closure. All this, of course, creates a distinct and often dramatic change in family dynamics. This chapter examines why and when people die. The following chapters continue by examining where and how people die.

HISTORICAL PERSPECTIVE

During its formative years, the United States largely was composed of agrarian, extended families. Most folks were self-reliant. The large agrarian and farming population frequently witnessed the birth and death of people as well as farm animals. Death was an expected and, for the most part, a natural event. In addition, because families were large and extended, everyone had some experience with someone who had recently died or was dying. The old and sick often were cared for at home by family members. There were farm or industrial accidents; bouts of diseases such as typhoid and yellow fever; flu epidemics; and childhood diseases such as measles, whooping cough, and diphtheria that resulted in numerous deaths. The Spanish influenza pandemic in 1918 caused by an avian H1N1 virus resulted in 50 million deaths worldwide (de Wit & Fouchier, 2008).

In the days before antibiotics, pneumonia was known as the "old person's friend" since pneumonia was the way many people passed on. Sulfa was the first antibiotic drug and came into use in the 1930s; penicillin came into use in 1943. Before the mid-20th century, the ill and dying mostly received palliative care.

This all changed during the second half of the 20th century, when technology boomed. Every year there were new medical discoveries and health care inventions. The sick, old, and terminally ill people fled from the simpler care of yesterday into the outstretched arms of the fully equipped intensive care unit. The era of the natural death was ushered out the door just like the custom of hanging laundry on a line in the yard. The intensive care hospital unit and the automatic dryer replaced the old expectations and the old ways. In only a few decades the whole tenor of the way people die changed.

As the agrarian period morphed into the industrial period and then into technological dominance, the era of the extended family also disappeared. Driven by new job opportunities, families moved apart and the social fabric of family support and strong individual self-reliance crumbled. By the end of the 20th century, the majority of old people spent the remainder of their days in nursing homes, kept alive much longer than in the generation before by innovative medical intervention. The irony is that the administrators of these new havens for the old and disabled did not want their records to reflect that their clientele died in-house, so when residents became gravely ill, an ambulance was summoned and the terminally ill, old person was transferred to an acute care facility. Here, faced with the life support paraphernalia of monitoring devices, IVs, and feeding tubes, many recovered and were returned to the nursing home. Those who did succumb in the hospital were quietly slipped down the back elevator and a demerit mark was put on the morbidity and mortality sheet of that particular service or attending physician. The fact that it might be natural to die was not in the picture and certainly not in the consciousness of the American psyche.

In the 1960s Dame Cicely Sanders, an English physician, came to the United States to introduce the concept of hospice for terminal cancer patients. It took the balance of the century for the model to finally take root and the practice of a peaceful death in a comfortable setting to become established. Despite the growth and acceptance of the hospice movement, the majority of the terminal elderly still suffer the indignities of acute hospital or nursing home care and end up dying in a foreign and painful setting.

WHY PEOPLE DIE

For most of human history, doctors and nurses could do little to cure most illnesses or extend human life. Those who lived to old age were considered most fortunate. Following the discovery of antibiotics and a plethora of other medications and technology, people began living longer and longer. Very few had the distinction of dying of old age or natural causes. These days almost every illness is clinically diagnosed, logged, and eventually recorded on the death certificate. Consequently, we have amassed a huge body of data called *vital statistics*.

In the United States, as in most developed countries, death is rarely unexpected. It usually occurs in older persons with chronic progressive illnesses that often are complicated by infections or exacerbations (Feeg & Elebiary, 2005). When analyzing and comparing the vital statistics and end stage illnesses and diseases of the past with those of today, we discover that life extension has resulted in many more chronic diseases, and now, many documented causes of death. Mortality data from the National Vital Statistics System are a fundamental source of demographic, geographic, and cause-of-death information. This is one of the few sources of health-related data that is comparable for geographic areas and available for a long period in the United States. The data are also used to present the characteristics of those dying in the United States, to determine life expectancy, and to compare mortality trends with other countries (Centers for Disease Control and Prevention, "National Vital Statistics System," n.d.). It is important to note that frequently there is a several–year lag between the time the data are gathered and the time when they are compiled, analyzed, and published. Hence the key mortality statistics presented here and in other data that follow are a few years old.

Deaths Worldwide

Table 1.1 shows the causes of reported human deaths worldwide in 2002 arranged by their associated mortality rates. Worldwide there were 57,029,000 deaths reported (about 58 million people). It is fascinating to look at this listing and see the range and scope of conditions from which people die.

The two leading causes of death in 2002 were cardiovascular disease (29%) and infectious parasitic diseases (23%). The third and fourth leading causes of death were ischemic heart disease (13%) and malignant neoplasms (12%).

Cancer as a Leading Cause of Death

Cancer is the leading cause of death worldwide in the year 2010. Low- and middle-income countries will experience the impact of higher can-

TABLE 1.1   World Deaths Per 100,000 Per Year in 2002

Cause of Death	Percentage of the whole
All causes	100.00
Cardiovascular diseases	29.34
Infectious and parasitic diseases	23.04
Ischemic heart disease	12.64
Malignant neoplasms (cancer)	12.49
Cerebrovascular disease (stroke)	9.66
Respiratory infections	6.95
Respiratory diseases	6.49
Unintentional injuries	6.49
HIV/AIDS	4.87
Chronic obstructive pulmonary disease	4.82
Perinatal conditions	4.32
Digestive diseases	3.45
Diarrheal diseases	3.15
Intentional injuries (suicide, violence, war)	2.84
Tuberculosis	2.75
Malaria	2.23
Lung cancers	2.18
Road traffic accidents	2.09
Childhood diseases	2.09
Neuropsychiatric disorders	1.95
Diabetes mellitus	1.73
Hypertensive heart disease	1.60
Suicide	1.53
Stomach cancer	1.49
Genitourinary system diseases	1.53
Cirrhosis of the liver	1.38
Nephritis/nephropathy	1.19
Colorectal cancer	1.09
Liver cancer	1.08
Measles	1.07

(Continued)

TABLE 1.1   (*Continued*)

Cause of Death	Percentage of the whole
Violence	0.98
Maternal conditions	0.89
Congenital abnormalities	0.86
Nutritional deficiencies	0.85
Breast cancer	0.84
Esophageal cancer	0.78
Inflammatory heart disease	0.71
Alzheimer's disease and dementias	0.70
Falls	0.69
Drowning	0.67
Poisoning	0.61
Lymphomas, multiple myeloma	0.59
Rheumatic heart disease	0.57
Oral and oropharynx cancers	0.56
Fires	0.55
Pertussis	0.52
Prostate cancer	0.47
Leukemia	0.46
Peptic ulcer disease	0.46
Protein-energy malnutrition	0.46
Endocrine/nutritional disorders	0.43
Asthma	0.42
Cervical cancer	0.42
Pancreatic cancer	0.41
Tetanus	0.38
Sexually transmitted diseases excluding HIV/AIDS	0.32
Bladder cancer	0.31
Meningitis	0.30
War	0.30
Syphilis	0.28

(*Continued*)

TABLE 1.1 *(Continued)*

Cause of Death	Percentage of the whole
Neoplasms other than malignant	0.26
Iron deficiency anemia	0.24
Ovarian cancer	0.24
Tropical diseases excluding malaria	0.23
Epilepsy	0.22
Musculoskeletal diseases	0.19
Hepatitis B	0.18
Parkinson's disease	0.17
Alcohol use disorders	0.16
Drug use disorders	0.15
Upper respiratory infections	0.13
Uterine cancer	0.12
Skin diseases	0.12
Melanoma and other skin cancers	0.12
Hepatitis C	0.09
Leishmaniasis	0.09
Trypanosomiasis	0.08
Benign prostatic hyperplasia	0.06

From "Annex Table 2: Deaths by cause, sex and mortality stratum in WHO regions, estimated for 2002," by World Health Organization, 2004, *The World Health Report 2004—Changing History*. Retrieved May 3, 2010, from http://www.who.int/entity/whr/2004/annex/topic/en/annex_2_en.pdf

cer incidence and death rates more sharply than industrialized countries.

Cases of cancer doubled globally between 1975 and 2000, will double again by 2020, and will nearly triple by 2030. There were an estimated 12 million new cancer diagnoses and more than 7 million deaths worldwide in 2009. The projected numbers for 2030 are 20 to 26 million new diagnoses and 13 to 17 million deaths. The global community can expect increases of incidence of about 1% each year, with larger increases in China, Russia, and India. Reasons for the increased rates include adoption of tobacco use and higher-fat diets in less-developed countries, and demographic changes, including a projected population increase of 38% in less-developed countries between 2008 and 2030 (Mulcahy, 2008). These statistics are in sharp contrast with another recent report (see the following) that shows that cancer incidence and death rates for men and women in the United States continue to decline.

United States

In contrast to the rest of the world, the United States has successfully combated most infections as well as waterborne and contagious diseases. In addition, advances in diagnoses and treatments have resulted in an expanded life span for most Americans. Exhibit 1.1 details the overall death and life expectancy data for the United States for 2006, the most recent data compiled.

Exhibit 1.2 details the fact that in 2006 most United States residents died primarily from five major processes: heart disease, cancer, stroke, chronic respiratory diseases, and accidents. The five secondary causes are diabetes, Alzheimer's disease, influenza and pneumonia, kidney diseases, and septicemia.

Figure 1.1 details the leading causes of death in graph form, while Figure 1.2 breaks the data down into age groups.

Note in Figure 1.1 that over 30% of the deaths in the 16- to 24-year-old category resulted from motor vehicle accidents. In the 55- to 64-year-old category just less than 40% of deaths were related to malignant neoplasms, a diagnosis that decreases relative to increasing age. Over 50% of deaths in the 85-and-older category were related to major cardiovascular diseases. There was no category for old age or natural deaths.

EXHIBIT 1.1   United States Deaths and Mortality, 2006

- Number of deaths: 2,426,264
- Death rate: 810.4 deaths per 100,000 population
- Life expectancy: 77.7 years
- Infant mortality rate: 6.69 deaths per 1,000 live births

From "Fast stats. Deaths and mortality. Final data for 2006, Tables B, D, 7, 30," by Centers for Disease Control and Prevention, 2010. Retrieved July 14, 2010, from http://www.cdc.gov/nchs/fastats/deaths.htm

EXHIBIT 1.2   Number of Leading Causes of Death in the United States, 2006

- Heart disease: 631,636
- Cancer: 559,888
- Stroke (cerebrovascular diseases): 137,119
- Chronic lower respiratory diseases: 124,583
- Accidents (unintentional injuries): 121,599
- Diabetes: 72,449
- Alzheimer's disease: 72,432
- Influenza and pneumonia: 56,326
- Nephritis, nephrotic syndrome, and nephrosis: 45,344
- Septicemia: 34,234

From "Fast stats. Deaths and mortality. Final data for 2006, Tables B, D, 7, 30," by Centers for Disease Control and Prevention, 2010. Retrieved July 14, 2010, from http://www.cdc.gov/nchs/fastats/deaths.htm

FIGURE 1.1   Leading causes of death in the United States in 2002.

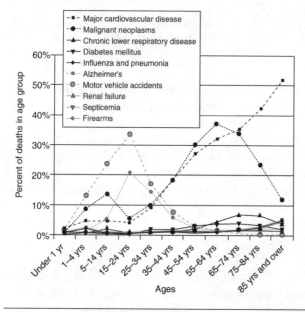

From "List of Causes of Death by Rate and Number: United States," by National Vital Statistics Report, 2002, *National Vital Statistics, 50* (15). Retrieved May 3, 2010, from http://en.wikipedia.org/wiki/List_of_causes_of_death_by_rate#United_States

FIGURE 1.2   Death in the United States by age group in 2002.

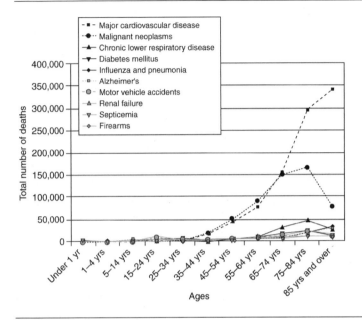

From "List of Causes of Death by Rate and Number: United States," by National Vital Statistics Report, 2002, *National Vital Statistics, 50*(15). Retrieved May 3, 2010, from http://en.wikipedia.org/wiki/List_of_causes_of_death_by_rate#United_States

In Figure 1.1, although cardiovascular disease begins a steep increase with the 55- to 64-year-old category, malignant neoplasms mirror this increase until the 65- to 74-year-old category and then begin to decline.

Figure 1.3 details the number and rate of fatal occupational injuries, by industry sector, in 2006 in the United States. In Figure 1.3 the four leading occupations in fatalities were construction; transportation and warehousing; agriculture, forestry, fishing, and hunting; and government.

Cancer

According to the American Cancer Society, cancer incidence and mortality rates in the United States are declining. The steady decline over the past 15 years means that about 650,000 deaths have been prevented or delayed. Nevertheless, cancer remains a leading cause of death, coming second after cardiovascular disease in 2006. The numbers are

FIGURE 1.3 Death rates by occupation in 2006.

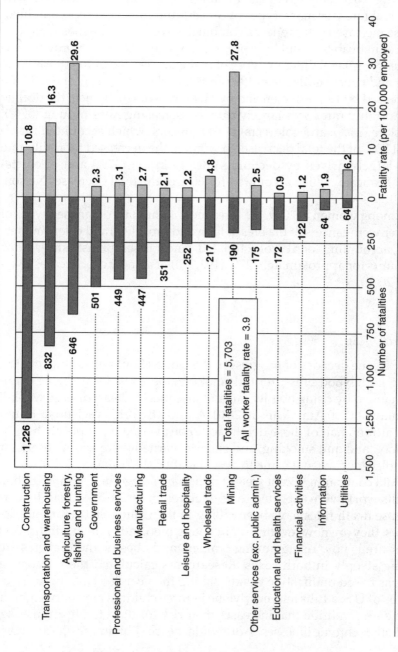

	Number of fatalities	Fatality rate (per 100,000 employed)
Construction	1,226	10.8
Transportation and warehousing	832	16.3
Agriculture, forestry, fishing, and hunting	646	29.6
Government	501	2.3
Professional and business services	449	3.1
Manufacturing	447	2.7
Retail trade	351	2.1
Leisure and hospitality	252	2.2
Wholesale trade	217	4.8
Mining	190	27.8
Other services (exc. public admin.)	175	2.5
Educational and health services	172	0.9
Financial activities	122	1.2
Information	64	1.9
Utilities	64	6.2

Total fatalities = 5,703
All worker fatality rate = 3.9

Source: From "National Census of Fatal Occupational Injuries in 2006," by the United States Department of Labor, Bureau of Labor Statistics, 2006, p. 4. Retrieved from http://www.bls.gov/news.release/archives/cfoi_08092007.pdf

still huge, with a total of about 1,500,000 new cancer cases a year (Nelson, 2009).

Since 1975, there have been notable improvements in relative 5-year survival rates for many types of cancers and for all cancers combined. These increased rates reflect a combination of earlier diagnoses and advances in treatment. But little progress has been made in improving outcomes for several different types of malignancies, including those of the lung and pancreas. Between 1990 and 2005, the overall cancer death rate decreased by 19.2% in men and by 11.4% in women. In men, the decline in mortality rates was largely due to decreasing rates of lung (37%), prostate (24%), and colorectal (17%) cancers, which accounted for almost 80% of the total decrease. In women, the decreased mortality rate was largely driven by declining rates in breast (37%) and colorectal (24%) cancers, which accounted for 60% of the total decrease (Nelson, 2009).

Among women in 2009, the three most commonly diagnosed types of cancer were cancers of the breast, lung and bronchus, and colon and rectum, accounting for 51% of estimated cancer cases. Breast cancer alone accounts for approximately 27% (192,370) of all new cancer cases (Nelson, 2009).

Heart Disease

Despite the decades of progress in the United States on cutting cholesterol, high blood pressure, and smoking, these results are being countermanded by rising obesity rates. Consequently, heart disease will kill around 400,000 Americans in 2010. A study by British scientists found that around half of those deaths could be averted if people ate healthier food and quit smoking, and experts warned there was no room for complacency when it came to heart health risks (Killand, 2010).

Data confirming recent weight trends are staggering, with 1.5 billion adults worldwide expected to be overweight by 2015. Although heart disease death rates have been falling in the United States for four decades, they are now leveling off in young men and women. High blood pressure is now rising among women, and obesity and diabetes are rising steeply in both sexes. Researchers calculated the number of deaths based on lifestyle trends, taking the year 2000 as a base. Two-thirds of U.S. adults and nearly one in three children are overweight or obese—a condition that increases their risk for diabetes, heart disease, and other chronic illnesses. Worldwide, nearly 1 billion adults are overweight and, if no action is taken, this figure will surpass 1.5 billion by 2015 (Killand, 2010).

SUMMARY

Knowing some of the statistics and having a better understanding of the causes of death perhaps makes it easier to appreciate that death is a natural part of the life cycle. In one way or another death comes to everyone. It comes through accident or disease and none us can avoid the inevitable.

With the contemporary unfolding of topics once taboo (sex, money, and politics), it seems timely to openly discuss the why, when, and wherefores of death. Death comes to all of us in some way. Likely it is easier to deal with death the more we recognize it in its many cloaks and colors.

Words of Wisdom

An ounce of prevention is worth a pound of cure.

[E]verything appears to promise that it will last; but in this world nothing is certain but death and taxes.
—Benjamin Franklin, 1706–1790

REFERENCES

Centers for Disease Control and Prevention. (2010). *Fast stats. Deaths and mortality. Final data for 2006, Tables B, D, 7, 30.* Retrieved July 14, 2010, from http://www.cdc.gov/nchs/fastats/deaths.htm

Centers for Disease Control and Prevention. (n.d.). *National Vital Statistics.* Retrieved August 18, 2010, from www.cdc.gov/nchs/nuss.htm

de Wit, E., & Fouchier, R. A. (2008). Emerging influenza. *Journal of Clinical Virology, 41*(1), 1–6.

Feeg, V. D., & Elebiary, H. (2005). Exploratory study on end-of-life issues: Barriers to palliative care and advance directives. *American Journal of Palliative Care, 22*(2), 119–124.

Killand, K. (2010). Heart disease will kill 400,000 Americans in 2010. In J. Lawrence (Ed.), *Reuters online newsletter.* Retrieved April 20, 2010, from http://www.reuters.com/article/idUSTRE6103EN20100201

Mulcahy, N. (2008, December 10). Cancer to become leading cause of death worldwide. *Medscape Medical News*. Retrieved May 3, 2010, from http://www.medscape.com/viewarticle/585098

National Vital Statistics Report. (2002, September 16). List of causes of death by rate and number: United States. *National Vital Statistics, 50*(15). Retrieved May 3, 2010, from http://en.wikipedia.org/wiki/List_of_causes_of_death_by_rate#United_States

Nelson, R. (2009, May 27). Cancer incidence and mortality rates declining in US. *Medscape Medical News Center*. Retrieved April 30, 2010, from http://www.medscape.com/viewarticle/703383

United States Department of Labor, Bureau of Labor Statistics. (2006). *National Census of Fatal Occupational Injuries in 2006*. Retrieved from http://www.bls.gov/news.release/archives/cfoi_08092007.pdf

World Health Organization. (2004). Annex Table 2: Deaths by cause, sex and mortality stratum in WHO regions, estimated for 2002. *The World Health Report 2004—Changing History*. Retrieved May 3, 2010, from http://www.who.int/entity/whr/2004/annex/topic/en/annex_2_en.pdf

2 *Death with Dignity*

Death is not the worst evil, but rather when we wish to die and cannot.

—Sophocles (ca. 496 B.C.–406 B.C.)

ANNA'S STORY   Anna W. was 90. She lived with her husband in their home of over 40 years. She been legally blind for over a decade but had the good fortune to survive two multimonth stays in nursing homes after suffering two broken hips and a broken pelvis.

At a recent, routine office visit she told her family practice doctor that she had been having increasing difficulty with bowel movements and had black, tarry stools. She asked what could be done. He replied, "Likely nothing. Would you want us to remove your colon if there were a problem?" He prescribed a laxative and stool softener. After that response, she sought counsel from her nurse daughter. She asked her daughter, "What is my prognosis?" Anna's daughter advised her to seek a gastrointestinal (GI) consult with a likely diagnostic CAT scan. Her daughter realized that bowel obstructions, from whatever source, can, and often do, present as an acute abdomen in the emergency department. Then emergency action is taken; little choice is offered for decision making when a patient is in acute pain. Surgery is the intervention of choice when a patient presents as a bowel obstruction emergency.

The GI doctor did the CAT scan and found that Anna did have Stage 4 metastatic bowel cancer. The options were a bowel resection with colostomy bag or referral to hospice. Following a family council considering all the options, Anna chose the hospice. Hospice attended Anna, made her comfortable, and gave the supporting analgesics during the eventual obstruction. Anna died at home with her family around her.

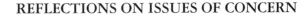

REFLECTIONS ON ISSUES OF CONCERN

1. When should attempts at medical diagnoses end?
2. Should a patient and his or her family be able to make pre-emptive choices?
3. Should there be a cutoff age after which diagnostic CAT scans are no longer offered?
4. Is it worth the cost(s) of diagnostic testing after a certain age if that testing renders the patient and family able to make more individualized decisions?
5. What are other variables that assist people with the opportunity for death with dignity?

AGING IN AMERICA

The U.S. population is rapidly aging. By 2030, the number of Americans age 65 and older will more than double to 71 million older Americans, comprising roughly 20% of the U.S. population. In some states, fully a quarter of the population will be age 65 and older. The cost of providing health care for an older American is three to five times greater than the cost for someone younger than 65. By 2030, the nation's health care spending is projected to increase by 25% due to demographic shifts unless improving and preserving the health of older adults is more actively addressed.

The State of Aging and Health in America (2007) report presents the most current national data available on 15 key health indicators for older adults related to health status, health behaviors, preventive care and screening, and injuries. The "State-by-State Report Card" provides similar information for each of the 50 states and the District of Columbia, and enables states to see where they are on each indicator as well as in relation to other states. The report includes "Calls to Action" and a "Spotlight" on reducing injuries associated with falls. These features highlight model intervention programs and thoughtful recommendations for policymakers, health care providers, and older adults themselves to ensure not just longer but healthier lives. Emerging public health opportunities include promoting cognitive health and addressing end-of-life decision-making issues (*The State of Aging and Health in America*, 2007).

Insurance company data on the elderly population describe the facts in a slightly different manner:

EXHIBIT 2.1   Data on Nursing Home Providers in the United States

1,813,665 total nursing facility beds
16,995 total nursing facilities
13% of facilities are hospital-based
52% of facilities are part of a chain
35% of facilities are individually owned and operated

Source: http://www.efmoody.com/longterm/nursingstatistics.html

Ages 65–74 make up 7% (18,759,000 people) of the total population.
Ages 75–84 make up 4% (11,145,000 people) of the total population.
Ages 85 and older make up 1% (3,625,000 people) of the total population.
The total elderly population age 65 and older makes up 13% of the total U.S. population.

Swelling numbers of these elderly end up in nursing homes and, as it turns out, the Medicare and Medicaid programs fund the majority of nursing home services. Medicare long-term care services are covered by Part A, "Skilled Nursing Facility" services, which are associated with postoperative or posthospitalization therapies, including rehabilitation. However, when posthospitalization coverage runs out, generally after three months, private insurance or personal pay then kicks in. The other coverage, by Medicaid (paid for by the state) "Nursing Facility" services, is provided to state residents who meet the Medicaid eligibility requirements. Exhibit 2.1 provides data on nursing home providers in the United States. Note that just over half (52%) of nursing home providers are part of a chain and are owned or leased by a multifacility organization.

These data yield insight into the plight of the old, terminally ill. Many are in nursing homes, on state aid, and without family. For these unfortunate ones, but also for those who do have relatives, this book details a place for death with dignity.

END-OF-LIFE PREPAREDNESS

Public health organizations have long rallied to address the overall health of the nation. It is noteworthy that they now address concerns for the end of life. Exhibit 2.2 details three characteristics of public health priorities at the end of life: "high burden, major impact, and a potential for preventing the suffering associated with illness."

Public health strategies, coupled with medical advances, have resulted in a marked 30-year increase in life expectancy since the beginning of the 20th century. In the past, most public health efforts focused on ensuring that infants had a healthy start in life and that children thrived and were protected from injury and infectious diseases. As people began living longer, their expectations about their health and the quality of their lives began increasing. Because of this phenomenon, attention focused on adults to engage them in healthy behaviors and take advantage of preventive measures that reduce the risk of chronic disease, injury, and infectious diseases such as influenza and pneumonia. Recently, expectations have evolved to wanting to ensure that the last months and days of life are lived as fully as possible, as pain-free as possible, and with dignity and choice. Thus, now, in addition to focusing on the beginning of life and continued good health throughout life, the Centers for Disease Control are extending their focus to life's close. Planning for the end of life is increasingly viewed as a public health issue given its potential to prevent unnecessary suffering and to support an individual's decisions and preferences related to the end of life (Centers for Disease Control and Prevention, 2010).

EXHIBIT 2.2   Point of View

"Public health activities to prevent and control disease have produced an extraordinary decline in mortality rates during the last century. This phenomenon has widespread implications, not the least of which is that death often occurs at a later age and frequently after a protracted illness. With a prolonged death due to technological advances now common in developed countries, quality of life at the end of life has become a societal concern. It is logical that public health should embrace the end of life as an area worthy of study and intervention. **After all, the end of life has three characteristics of other public health priorities: high burden, major impact, and a potential for preventing the suffering associated with illness.**"

From Rao, Anderson, and Smith, (2002, p. 215).

Preparing for Transition

Not all family caregivers are adept at assisting their loved ones in passing. As Exhibit 2.3 shows, most are unprepared for the death of their loved one. In this instance researchers outlined certain factors that fam-

EXHIBIT 2.3   Research Perspective

Many family caregivers are unprepared for the death of their loved one and may suffer from deteriorating mental health as a result. Because of this premise a group of researchers sought to determine the factors that family caregivers believe are important to preparing for death and bereavement. Focus groups and ethnographic interviews were conducted with 33 family caregivers (bereaved or current) of terminally ill patients. Life experiences such as the duration of caregiving/illness, advance care planning, previous experiences with caregiving or death, and medical sophistication all impacted preparedness, or the degree to which a caregiver is ready for the death and bereavement.

- Regardless of life experiences all caregivers reported medical, practical, psychosocial, and religious/spiritual uncertainty.
- Because uncertainty was multidimensional, caregivers often needed more than prognostic information in order to prepare.
- Communication was the primary mechanism used to manage uncertainty. Good communication included clear, reliable information, combined with relationship-centered care from health care providers.
- Finally, preparedness had cognitive, affective, and behavioral dimensions. To prepare, some caregivers needed information tailored to their uncertainty (cognitive), others needed to mentally or emotionally prepare (affective), and still others had important tasks to complete (behavioral).

To better prepare family caregivers for the death of a loved one, health care providers must develop a trusting relationship with caregivers, provide them with reliable information tailored to their uncertainty, and allow time for caregivers to process the information and complete important tasks.

From Hebert, Schulz, Copeland, and Arnold (2009).

ily caregivers believe are important to preparing for death and bereavement. Prolific author and gerontological nurse leader Charlotte Eliopoulos (2005, 2009) advocates for nurses to gain as much information as possible in order to provide the kind and scope of care that is needed for our old and increasingly older population.

DEATH WITH DIGNITY

The greatest human freedom is to live and die according to one's own desires and beliefs. The most common desire among those with a terminal disease is to die with some measure of dignity. From advance directives to physician-assisted dying, death with dignity is a movement to provide options for the dying to control their own end-of-life care (Death with Dignity National Center, 2010). Advance directives allow individuals to communicate in advance their desires for end-of-life care. Although the statutes vary from state to state, advance directives are a step in the right direction. As such they are an excellent place for individuals to state their preference for a place for death with dignity: the *Golden Room* for end-of-life care.

ADVANCE DIRECTIVES

What kind of medical care would you want for yourself or your loved ones if you or they were too ill or hurt to express final wishes? For example, if you were in a coma or serious car wreck and were admitted to the hospital, hospital staff would inquire about advance directives. Advance directives are legal documents that convey one's end-of-life decisions ahead of time. They provide a way to communicate one's wishes to family, friends, and health care professionals and to avoid confusion later on. Advance directives can take many forms. Laws about advance directives are different in each state. Those writing an advance directive should be aware of the laws in their own state.

A good advance directive describes the kind of treatment you would want depending on how sick you are. For example, the directive would describe what kind of care you want if you have an illness that you are unlikely to recover from or if you are permanently unconscious. Advance directives usually detail that you don't want certain kinds of treatment, such as resuscitation. However, they can also say that you want a certain treatment no matter how ill you are.

Writing an Advance Directive

Advance directives and living wills do not have to be complicated legal documents. They can be short, simple statements about what you want done or not done if you cannot speak for yourself. It is important to note that anything you write by yourself or with a computer software package should follow your state laws. You may also want to have your physician or lawyer review what you have written to make sure your directives are understood exactly as you intended. When you are satisfied with your directives, the orders should be notarized if possible, and copies should be given to your family and your doctor.

You can write an advance directive in several ways:

- Use the form provided by your doctor or hospital upon admission.
- Write your wishes down yourself and carry them with you. You may even use a computer software package for legal documents.
- Call your health department or state department on aging to request an advance directive form.
- Work with an attorney to create an advance directive that reflects your own wishes.

Advantages of Advance Directives

By creating an advance directive, one makes preferences about medical care known before being faced with a serious injury or illness. This can spare loved ones the stress of making decisions about care during a crisis. For example, someone with terminal cancer might write that he or she does not want to be on a respirator if he or she stops breathing. This action can reduce suffering, increase peace of mind, and increase control over one's own destiny. Any person 18 years of age or older can prepare an advance directive. Even when in good health, it is a good idea to write an advance directive. An accident or serious illness can happen suddenly, and if one already has a signed advance directive, one's wishes are more likely to be followed.

Changing Advance Directives

An individual can change or cancel an advance directive at any time, as long as the individual is considered to be of sound mind. Being of sound mind means that the person is still able to think rationally and communicate wishes in a clear manner. The changes must be made, signed, and notarized according to the laws in the specific state. Make sure that your caregivers and any family members who knew about the directives are also aware that have been changed.

When there is no time to put changes in writing, the person can make them known while hospitalized. The person should inform the doctor and any family or friends present exactly what he or she wants to happen. Usually, wishes that are made in person will be followed in place of the ones made earlier in writing. Be sure the instructions are clearly understood by everyone being told.

Living Will

A living will is one type of advance directive. It is a written, legal document that describes the kind of medical treatments or life-sustaining treatments you want if seriously or terminally ill. A living will does not let you select someone to make decisions for you. By use of a living will one can accept or refuse medical care. There are many end-of-life issues to consider, including

- The use of dialysis and breathing machines
- Insertion or use of tube feeding
- Cardiac resuscitation
- Organ or tissue donation

Durable Power of Attorney

A durable power of attorney (DPA) for health care is another kind of advance directive. It is a document that names a health care proxy. A proxy is someone who is trusted to make health decisions if the patient is unable to do so. A DPA states the person chosen to make health care decisions for the patient. It becomes active any time the patient is unconscious or unable to make medical decisions. A DPA is generally more useful than a living will. However, a DPA may not be a good choice for patients who do not have another person they trust to make these decisions for them.

Living wills and DPAs are legal in most states. Even if they are not officially recognized by the law in your state, they can still guide loved ones and doctors if and when patients are unable to make decisions about their own medical care.

Do Not Resuscitate

A Do Not Resuscitate (DNR) order is another kind of advance directive. A DNR is a request not to have cardiopulmonary resuscitation (CPR) during cardiac arrest or if you stop breathing. Without a DNR in your record, hospital staff will generally move to resuscitation. One can use an advance directive form or tell one's doctor that one does not want to be resuscitated. When one signs this form, a DNR order is put in one's medical chart and usually is prominent in the person's room, often at the head of the bed.

Planning for care at the end of life can make things easier for people as they die and reduce stress and depression among loved ones. With advance care planning, people have the opportunity to declare how they would like to be treated at the end of their lives. They can pinpoint the kinds of medical and resuscitation services they prefer and appoint people to serve as their surrogate decision makers.

OTHER OPTIONS FOR DEATH WITH DIGNITY

In the past couple of decades many have paid attention to other end-of-life options. Strides for death with dignity appear to be happening slowly, yet they are being made and the momentum has been gradually building.

Death with Dignity National Action Centers

The Death with Dignity National Center (DDNC) is the leader in this movement, successfully establishing, advancing, and defending the landmark Oregon Death with Dignity Act, and is a national catalyst for openly discussing and actively reforming end-of-life care for those who are terminally ill (Death with Dignity National Center, 2010).

The Hemlock Society

The Hemlock Society was founded by Derek Humphry in 1980 and became the largest and oldest right-to-die organization in America. This organization fought for voluntary euthanasia and physician-assisted suicide to be made legal for terminally and hopelessly ill adults. Hemlock's principles were to:

- Educate and advise dying people on how to bring about a peaceful end when dying; trapped in a ruined body; or simply terminally old, frail, and tired of life.
- Give aid through specialized literature and moral support. The organization never provided hands-on assistance in dying to people because it needed to stay within the law.
- Draft and launch the first model law governing euthanasia and assisted suicide in America, in 1986, from which many others that were to follow were refined.
- Financially and physically back referenda in California, Washington State, Michigan, Oregon, and Maine.
- Found and launch a national "Caring Friends" program so that maximum personal support and assistance in dying, within the law, could be ensured to every member.
- Produce the book *Final Exit*, which detailed exactly how to carry out this final passage. (Humphry, 2005)

Compassion & Choices

In 2003, the Hemlock Society morphed into a new organization, Compassion & Choices. This nonprofit organization works to improve care and expand choice at the end of life. As a national organization with over 60 local groups, affiliates, and chapters and 30,000 members, this group helps patients and their loved ones face the end of life with calming facts and choices of action during a difficult time. It also aggressively pursues legal reform to promote pain care, fight for advance directives, and legalize physician aid in dying (*Compassion and Choices*, n.d.).

Death with Dignity Acts

The Northwest appears to be leading the way with specific state legislation regarding death with dignity. First Oregon in 1997, and then Washington in 2008, accepted death with dignity and laid down specific criteria.

Oregon

Oregon voters changed the entire debate about end-of-life care. After surviving repeal efforts, legal challenges that went all the way to the Supreme Court, and efforts by the Bush administration to shut down the law, Oregon residents voted to sustain their plea. On October 27, 1997, Oregon enacted the Death with Dignity Act, which allows terminally ill

Oregonians to end their lives through the voluntary self-administration of lethal medications, expressly prescribed by a physician for that purpose.

The act was a citizens' initiative that Oregon voters passed twice. The first time was in a general election in November 1994, when it passed by a margin of 51% to 49%. An injunction delayed implementation of the act but was lifted on October 27, 1997. In November 1997, a measure was placed on the general election ballot to repeal the act. Voters chose to retain the act by a margin of 60% to 40%.

There is no state program for participation in the act, nor do people apply to the State of Oregon or the Department of Human Services. It is up to qualified patients and licensed physicians to implement the act on an individual basis. The act does require the Oregon Department of Human Services to collect information about the patients and physicians who participate in the act and to publish an annual statistical report.

The law states that, in order to participate, a patient must be (1) 18 years of age or older, (2) a resident of Oregon, (3) capable of making and communicating health care decisions for himself or herself, and (4) diagnosed with a terminal illness that will lead to death within six months. The attending physician determines whether these criteria have been met. The Oregon experience shows that the aid-in-dying law benefits all at the end of life, provides comfort and control to the terminally ill, and ends violent deaths (*Oregon Government, Death with Dignity Act*, n.d.).

Washington

On November 4, 2008, Washington State became the second state to legalize aid in dying. Voters of Washington stood up for the rights of terminally ill individuals and passed the Washington Death with Dignity Act 59% to 41%. The passage of Washington's I-100 is considered a turning point on the path to human liberty. The people of Washington opted for individual liberty, personal autonomy, and freedom of conscience (Death with Dignity National Center, 2010).

Words of Wisdom

"Terminal care is an important phase of life, one in which individuals have the right to expect quality of care to ensure that their death occurs with dignity."

From Barham (2003).

CONSIDERING RESOURCES

The nation's current economic crisis makes addressing health care issues even more urgent. With health care spending on track to reach 50% of America's gross domestic product by 2050 and states in severe budgetary straits, cutting waste and creating new and innovative improvements to achieve savings while providing better care are imperative. Incremental change isn't enough. Groups are working together now to take immediate action to transform our system.

Some demographics project birth rates falling and life spans continuing to lengthen over the next two decades, driving up the median ages in many countries. The United States is now passing through an important demographic transition. Public discussion about the impact of this transition focuses primarily on how the aging population—and, in particular, the imminent retirement of the sizable baby boomer generation—will further lower the already-dismal national savings. This discussion often ignores additional important and potent demographic forces, including the behavioral differences in savings patterns between baby boomers and subsequent generations, the reduction in the birth rate, and the impact of the demographic transition already underway in many of the world's most important economies. In the past, the aging of the baby boomers supported wealth accumulation as they moved through their peak income and saving years, but this was recently overwhelmed by strong behavioral trends to save less. Now, baby boomers' entry into retirement will reinforce these behavioral trends to create a significant financial headwind. Boomers will save less, younger generations will continue to save less, and birth rates will slow. The resulting decline in the rate of wealth accumulation means less household savings will be available to support a fast-growing retiree and indigent population. At the same time, it will become increasingly difficult to support domestic investment and sustain economic growth (McKinsey Global Institute Demographics, n.d.).

POPULATION PROJECTIONS

Based on current projections, the U.S. population is expected to increase to 392 million by 2050—more than a 50% increase from the 1990 population size (McKinsey Global Institute Demographics, n.d.). The U.S. population will be older than it is now according to most projection series. The median age of the population will steadily increase to about 39 years old in 2035 and then level off. This increasing median age is driven by the aging of the population born during the baby boom after World War II (1946 to 1964). About 30% of the population in 1994 was born during the baby boom. As this group ages, the median age will rise. People born during the baby boom years were between 36 and 54 years old at the turn of the century. In 2011, the first members of the baby boom will reach age 65 while the baby boomers will have decreased to 25% of the total population. The last of the baby boom population will reach age 65 in the year 2029. By that time, the boomers are projected to be only about 16% of the total population. The mean life expectancy is anticipated to increase from 76.0 years in 1993 to 82.6 years in 2050. In 2050, life expectancy would range from 75.3 years to 87.5 years (U.S. Census Bureau, *Population Profile*, n.d.).

In 2030, when all of the baby boomers will be 65 and older, nearly one in five U.S. residents is expected to be 65 and older. This age group is projected to increase to 88.5 million in 2050, more than double the number in 2008 (38.7 million). Similarly, the 85-and-older population is expected to more than triple, from 5.4 million to 19 million, between 2008 and 2050 (U.S. Census Bureau, *Population*, n.d.; Centers for Disease Control and Prevention, n.d.).

CONSEQUENCES FOR OUR SOCIETY

Today we are faced with dire-sounding predictions from all directions, with required action that needed to happen yesterday. Where do we begin and how? There are many things that we cannot do anything about, such as our personal aging and death. There are also things that we can change, such as the care and quality of our dying experience.

We are entering a time of great change on all levels, similar to the yin and yang symbol that suggests both danger and opportunity. The danger is in doing nothing, being fearful and stagnant and feeling helpless. It is in allowing things to happen to us instead of through us. The opportunity is in taking bold, new, out-of-the-box steps to begin to change what is not working. Each heartfelt step, large or small, is a step toward solutions.

To meet the impending challenges, the authors envision a place called the *Golden Room*. Here patients would receive an alternative to enhance the quality of the death experience for both those dying and their families. In difficult times it is personal relationships that encourage and support us. To be part of the solution means taking a stand and getting involved in what opens our heart. Are we part of the problem by complaining or part of the solution by taking the first steps?

SUMMARY

With all the advance directives and other options for death with dignity that are available it would appear that Americans have a smorgasbord of choices, and yet the majority of the elderly die alone in acute care settings or nursing homes. It is time to make dying sacred and return it to its place of importance along with birth. All the directives in the world are useless if they are not honored. Imagine how you want to die. Will all your advance directives be sufficient if your family and caregivers are not comfortable with death and dying? Where is the honor and dignity in that?

The Golden Room described in Chapter 3 offers a beautiful, dignified place for the end-of-life transition. This special place offer a depth and scope of care that can transform, for the dying person and the family, the suffering of life's final phase into a cushioned, caring, more gentle passage into the unseen but ever-calling future.

REFERENCES

Barham, D. (2003). The last 48 hours of life: A case study of symptom control for a patient taking a Buddhist approach to dying. *International Journal of Palliative Nursing, 9*(6), 245–251.

Centers for Disease Control and Prevention. (2010). *End of life preparedness—An emerging public health priority.* Retrieved May 3, 2010, from http://www.cdc.gov/aging/endoflife/index.htm

Centers for Disease Control and Prevention. (n.d.) *Aging.* Retrieved May 3, 2010, from http://www.cdc.gov/Aging/EOL.html

Compassion and choices: Choice and care at the end of life. (n.d.). Retrieved May 3, 2010, from http://www.compassionandchoices.org/

Death with Dignity National Center. (2010). Retrieved May 3, 2010, from http://www.deathwithdignity.org/

Eliopoulos, C. (2005). New educational opportunities to improve competencies in geriatric care. *Beginnings, 25*(5), 8–9.

Eliopoulos, C. (2009). *Gerontological nursing.* Philadelphia: Lippincott Williams & Wilkins.

Hebert, R. S., Schulz, R., Copeland, V. C., & Arnold, R. M. (2009). Preparing family caregivers for death and bereavement. Insights from caregivers of terminally ill patients. *Journal of Pain Symptom Management, 37*(1), 3–12.

Humphry, D. (2005). *Farewell to Hemlock: Killed by its name. Euthanasia, research and guidance organization.* Retrieved April 30, 2010, from http://www.assistedsuicide.org/farewell-to-hemlock.html

McKinsey Global Institute Demographics. Retrieved May 3, 2010, from http://www.mckinsey.com/mgi/publications/demographics/index.asp

Oregon Government, Death with Dignity Act. (n.d.) Retrieved May 3, 2010, from http://www.oregon.gov/DHS/ph/pas/

Rao, J. K., Anderson, L. A., & Smith, S. (2002). End of life is a public health issue. *American Journal of Preventative Medicine, 23*(3), 215–220.

The State of Aging and Health in America. (2007). Whitehouse Station, NJ: The Merck Company Foundation. Retrieved April 30, 2010, from www.cdc.gov/Aging/saha.htm

U.S. Census Bureau. (n.d.) *Population profile: National project.* Retrieved May 3, 2010, from http://www.census.gov/population/www/pop-profile/natproj.html

U.S. Census Bureau. (n.d.) *Population* [Press release]. Retrieved May 3, 2010, from http://www.census.gov/PressRelease/www/releases/archives/population/012496.html

http://www.efmoody.com/longterm/nursingstatistics.html

3 A Place for Death with Dignity: The Golden Room

I think one's feelings waste themselves in words. They ought all to be distilled into actions and into actions which bring results.
—Florence Nightingale

JESSE'S STORY   Jesse Rodriguez was a fisherman. For most of his life he cast his nets off the sandy shores of Yelapa, Mexico. Following the death of his wife, he moved to southern California to live with his daughter. He worked as a part-time landscaper there for about 10 years until he was 65 and complained of chest pain. He was diagnosed with cardiac insufficiency and a vascular stent was inserted. Over the next decade he puttered around playing checkers with the locals in the park. Attending his granddaughters' 15-year-old Quinceañero celebration was the highlight of those years.

Following his 80th birthday Jesse began having increasing episodes of angina. One Sunday night his daughter, son-in-law, and four grandchildren took Jesse to the local emergency room, which was not equipped for cardiac emergencies. Jesse was sent by ambulance to a regional medical center three hours away from home. Two days later, after the extended family arrived, the medical team prescribed a full quadruple heart bypass; Jesse went to surgery. He survived the operating room and the routine 24 hours in the cardiac intensive care unit (ICU) and then moved on to the post-op unit.

The family camped in the hallways and lingered in the cafeteria. Social service worked with them to generate funds for living expenses during their stay in the city. A translator was provided to accompany Jesse to various post-op testing, therapies, and evaluation appointments.

The third day in the post-op unit, Jesse developed severe diarrhea. Stool samples were taken, and 24 hours later the suspected diagnosis of Clostridium difficile (C. diff) was confirmed. An IV was restarted to administer high doses of antibiotics, but the diarrhea had taken its toll. Jesse felt very weak and discouraged. The following day, the diarrhea subsided just as the pseudomous wound infection at the chest surgery site was discovered. Discouraged in mind and body, Jesse declared this wasn't worth the fight. Despite the massive antibiotic therapy, he deteriorated. He refused to get out of bed and, seven posthospitalization days later, Jesse passed away. His doctors presented his case to the hospital morbidity and mortality monthly meeting to see how they might have better handled the situation to prevent his death.

REFLECTIONS ON ISSUES OF CONCERN

1. When in the course of one's lifetime might serious discussion about end-of-life decisions be initiated?
2. Would it be appropriate to develop an age range and other criteria for doing major surgery on the elderly?
3. What is the expected life expectancy for someone over age 80 who undergoes quadruple bypass surgery?
4. What percentage of patients over 80 suffer from complications?
5. What are the morbidity and mortality rates of elderly patients receiving major surgery?
6. Were there other options that might have been considered for Jesse's care?
7. How many health care dollars are available for intensive, invasive care for the elderly? Should we consider some sort of criteria for use of those dollars?
8. Might there have been a way for Jesse to have a more peaceful end?
9. Might there be somewhere else for Jesse to go to have a better end?

THE NEED FOR SOMETHING NEW

Without a doubt, modern science continues to devise methods and techniques to keep people alive longer than ever. With the prolongation of life and increasing sophistication of medicine and technology, how one dies is becoming increasing relevant for more and more people and their families. This is an issue that society and the government will address at some point. The idea of helping people die with dignity, without unnecessary suffering and humiliation, is critically important for each of us, for family members, and for those of us who care for the dying. As a culture and a society, we must decide when to stop prolonging a life that has lost all the pleasure and meaning of living or a life that is artificially extended. In this book, the *Golden Room* is proposed as a place where people can go to find solace and comfort in their final days of life.

THE GOLDEN ROOM: A SPECIAL PLACE TO BE

There are approximately 2,426,000 deaths per year in the United States (Centers for Disease Control and Prevention, 2009). It is time that we, as a society, pay more attention to where, when, why, and how we prepare for and deal with the end of life. Many souls are alone at their time of death. Who are they, you ask? You may think that everyone dies at home in the hands of a caring hospice team, but this is not the case. Countless hundreds reside in nursing homes and come to their end in a two-bed room on a nondescript hall in one of the thousands of nursing homes that dot every state in America. Others face death in the crowed room of their personal residence, generally accompanied by a family member. It is the lucky ones among these homebound persons who also have the care and attendance of a hospice worker and family member. Still others meet their end in the ICU of an acute care hospital amid the hustle and bustle of scurrying hospital personnel using a countless, never-ending supply of invasive measures to keep their patients alive just a little bit longer.

Is there an alternative? You bet there is. *The Golden Room* is a new concept of a place that offers a way to fulfill a pressing societal need, the need to provide for death with dignity. What, then, you likely ask, is a *Golden Room*? (See Exhibit 3.1.)

EXHIBIT 3.1   Point of View

Think of the word *golden*. What does this seemingly simple term conjure up in your mind?

- Golden eyes
- Rays of sunshine
- Fall leaves
- Sunsets
- Golden dreams
- Golden years
- Golden days
- Or maybe even a painted *golden room*

(Continued)

EXHIBIT 3.1   (*Continued*)

For each of us *golden* may have some special meaning; with a few more of us, the phrase *the golden room* may suggest something else. In this book, the *Golden Room* is the name of the place where people in transition between life and death can go along with their families and friends to experience their last time together and final good-byes. In this location they can make peace with themselves, their loved ones, and the world as it exists in their frame of reality. *The Golden Room* is a metaphor for a place where dying people can find comfort and solace as they prepare for their final big physical event—the ending of their physical life journey and the beginning of their journey beyond our understanding.

PHYSICAL DESCRIPTION

To begin, imagine a new space, a specially designed room just for dying, the *Golden Room* itself. You open the door from the hallway and walk into a full-sized, spacious room. Immediately you appreciate the clean aroma while you note the sensation of inhaling electronically enhanced, purified air. Instead of the customary blaring TV so common in most patient settings, you see a full-picture, wall-mounted screen with images of gentle sea creatures undulating through blue-green, foamy seawater. After a few minutes the sea-life scene morphs into a host of airborne birds and butterflies in various stages of gliding through pastoral meadows and fluffy, ever-changing cloud formations.

You note that the walls are covered with washable, sound-absorbent material that is a lovely golden color. There is a hospital bed on one side of the room, surrounded by tray tables and stands to support supplies, dinner trays, and other miscellaneous items. At the window there are damask drapes that open to allow full daylight in or close tightly with complete light-blocking backing to allow for the adjustment to whatever degree of light or darkness is desired.

The ceiling is designed and built with a tray style. In other words, along the four edges an 8- to 12-inch rim is dropped down to create the effect of framing the ceiling. This style is used in bedrooms and some dining rooms in many contemporary homes. The goal in this instance is to allow the framed-in primary expanse of the ceiling to be decorated with an ornate mural. From the position of the recumbent patient a full view of a painted scene is just above and beyond his or her bed. In

Golden Rooms the mural above may display one of several forms of the cosmos. Some rooms have pastel cloud formations, and others may be a dark blue background with bright stars pebbled throughout the expanse of space. The floor is wood laminate. It gives the feel of warmth but allows for thorough and easy daily cleaning.

In an alcove in one corner of the room there is another bed and a re-clining chair. It is partitioned away from the hospital bed with sliding, movable screens. This corner can accommodate two loved ones who want to stay on-site. A roomy bathroom serves both the patient and the family. Table 3.1 outlines details of the *Golden Room*.

Even the bedding is tailor-made for the *Golden Room*. Instead of the familiar white cotton sheets of general hospitals and nursing homes, soft flannel sheets cover the bed. Fitted bottom sheets offer superior

TABLE 3.1   The Golden Room Description

Characteristic	Description
Walls	Gold color, rich texture, sound-absorbing material
Flooring	Laminate wood; feeling of warmth, easy to clean
Windows	Open to light; full, dark, lining drapes to open or close at will
Ceiling	Tray ceilings with murals of heaven or cosmos
Wall coverings	Pastoral or beautiful landscape paintings in muted colors
Bathroom	Attached to room; can accommodate both patient and family.
Television	Channel selection includes program of ever-changing pastoral nature scenes; or can be used to play DVDs, with a selection of uplifting programs designed to soothe and comfort
Music	Comes through stereo on television or sound box by patient's bedside; selection of a variety of styles: classical, soft rock, country, jazz, and some ethnic selections such as Indian selections, etc.

comfort and better reduce the often-crinkly noise and creases of the still-necessary moisture-protection mattress pad. A comforter or favorite blanket from home tops the bedding.

MENTAL AND EMOTIONAL AMBIANCE

The Golden Room's physical environment exudes a sense of a place for rest and gentle being. Colors, fabrics, and décor are selected for their mood feelings of gentle peace, relaxation, insight, and rest. Unlike the basal daytime noise level of 80–120 dB in the hospital's ICU (Carvalho, Pedreira, & deAguiar, 2005), which is far above the recommended 45 dB, the *Golden Room* is quiet and calming with soothing music. In fact, the music selections act as a natural pacemaker and slow down the heart rate, brain waves, and respirations. Music thanatology is used. This field of music therapy focuses on care of the dying through the use of pre-scriptive music (Morris, 2009). As such, it assists the person to release the physical body during the final hours before death by augmenting peace, recognition, and calm expectation.

The soft, comfortable furniture designed for a homey feel reflects a feeling of snuggling in and being at ease. The dimmer switch on the lighting makes for easy, family-directed control of lighting. A side table lamp offers the option of adding additional colors of blues and purples, tones designed to relax and calm. The air may or may not have the gentle aroma of essential oils, as the person desires. The person simply needs to ask staff to initiate this additional element. All these embellishments offer ways for the patient and family to tone down the environment and create the right mix of calming options tailor made just for them.

SPIRITUAL TONE

The purpose of the *Golden Room* is to facilitate and honor the dying process, both for the patients and their loved ones. To create that place all elements of the design are taken into consideration. The physical room reflects calm and inclusion for all members present in the environment. Certain features designed into the space augment the sense of peace and security. A sense of spirit is reflected from the centerpiece ceiling mural. Scenes depicting the cosmos with ethereal themes draw the supine pa-tient below upward into a dimension of cosmic design. Some patients may sense a feeling of being drawn upward into their personal concep-tion of spirit. Others may not consciously relate to a star-studded mural or a painting of angels bursting from clouds, but subconsciously they will likely be relating to something much greater than themselves.

Specially trained staff who are themselves comfortable with the process of death and dying assist in setting the spiritual tone of the *Golden Room*. Being comfortable with their own mortality as well as this natural end-of-life process allows the staff to be fully present for the person and the family as they move through this transition phase of life. These staff are able to soothingly create close, gentle relationships with each patient and family member, which enhances the final transition for all present (Iranmanesh, Häggström, Axelsson, & Sävenstedt, 2009).

GOLDEN ROOMS: WHERE ARE THEY?

No doubt you are familiar with hospice and palliative care, but *Golden Rooms* offer a new concept. You have now read the description of the room itself, but you may wonder, Where are they? *Golden Rooms* may be free standing, on the same site as a health care facility but in separate dedicated buildings, or attached to existing health care centers.

Acute Care Settings

Most health care providers are conversant with acute care centers such as general and specialty hospitals, veterans care centers, and urgent care centers. Think about the ICU or coronary care unit you know best. Now realize that nearly half of all Americans who die in hospitals spend time in the ICU during their last 3 days of life (O'Mahony et al., 2010). In this same ICU location critically ill patients receive aggressive life-sustaining interventions, suffering is common, and death is expected in up to 20% of patients (Mularski et al., 2009). Then consider whether the dying might be transferred to a specially developed area of the hospital for their transition. Think about the advantage, both to the staff and to the patient, of a transfer to the *Golden Room*. Think about how many patients you have with no chance of recovery who continue to reside on your unit while they die.

Medical and surgical floors, likewise flooded with chronically ill, sometimes terminal patients, could dedicate a section in their units, depending on their in-house mortality statistics. A design team composed of nurses and administrators could plan the features and have the builder remodel an existing ordinary hospital room into the *Golden Room*. Then terminal patients with nowhere else to go would be transferred to the *Golden Room* for the last hours or days of life (see Chapter 12).

Nursing Homes

Data tell us that many elderly die in nursing homes. Nursing homes are the site of 20% to 25% of all deaths; data suggest the number will be closer to 50% by 2050. How hard would it be for these facilities to modify some area for dying purposes? Not hard at all. We desperately need dedicated, special support rooms for our mainly solitary nursing home residents. Even those lucky ones with family may have only another infirm spouse who comes to visit. Think of the improvement when that significant other is able to pay his or her last respects to a loved one who is being supported in an upgraded, lovely room with a specially trained, dedicated staff. It is time to change the whole culture of what it means to die with dignity.

Freestanding Centers

Although to date there are no freestanding centers with the specific name *Golden Room*, a few freestanding hospice centers very closely approximate the concept, the design, and the philosophy of care. Two examples may serve as role models for the expansion of the concept. One long-standing traditional facility in an old, remodeled building in Boca Raton, Florida, has managed to capture the essence of a very peaceful, natural environment and heart-centered end-of-life care. It has private rooms that open onto a shared central garden courtyard. As a contrast a brand-new, recently built freestanding building in Spokane, Washington, sought to utilize the best concepts of design space, including a central courtyard with access from each room, and fully actualized holistic end-of-life care. These two prototypes, one old but remodeled, another newly built, serve as magnificent examples of how we can design and create many freestanding end-of-life care centers.

PAIN MANAGEMENT

In the *Golden Room* pain management is paramount. Care is given to administer enough pharmaceutical medications to control pain but not an amount that would depress the patient's respiratory or neurological functions. Since many prefer that their IV be removed, medications are generally delivered by the nurse via the intact port-a-cath, or by mouth. On occasions, however, patients may have an IV patient-controlled analgesia pump so they can control their own level and amount of pain medication.

PASTORAL CARE

Patients and families in the *Golden Room* have ready access to pastoral care. Chaplains, priests, rabbis, and/or the minister or pastoral counselor of choice are available to both the patient and the family. Pastoral care offers spiritual comfort, words of peace, and gentle release from the mind's worries about one's life, accomplishments, relationships, and mortality.

The subtle discernment process within pastoral care at the end of life brings forth the unanswered questions that most people have thought about at some point in time. As the end of physical life approaches, many persons revisit these questions in a final attempt to bring meaning into their lives. Families oftentimes revisit these lifetime questions to assist their understanding of what their dying loved one has accomplished and to establish that this life has some degree of meaning/satisfaction and therefore closure. These questions deal with basic feelings or the sense one has made of one's life. This includes a sense of identity, a sense of community, a sense of one's life's work, and a sense of mortality. These questions are reflected in Table 3.2.

There is no hierarchy in these questions; instead, each usually moves into another one and another one. The answers can be quite exquisite as a rich tapestry or an ornate, intricate tree of life. Pastoral care at the end of life is often involved in dealing with all four of these questions simultaneously.

In the *Golden Room* the Shepherds of the Cloth assist both the dying and their families by being fully present and not providing shallow ready-made answers. Through this most loving and compassionate approach, the patient and family can find both the question and then the

TABLE 3.2   Senses of Life and Questions to Ponder

Life's Senses	Life's Questions
Identity	Who am I?
Community	Who is my family/community?
One's life's work	What is my contribution?
Mortality	What is my God?

answer for themselves and come to peace with all that was, all that is, and all that will be.

HEALING MODALITIES

Many healing modalities are available in the *Golden Room*. Attention to detail and the physical ambiance of the room are part of this concept. Also keenly important is the care and support of the dying person. In addition to pain management and pastoral care there are many hands-on modalities to enhance a peaceful and comfortable passing.

A host of complementary and integrative therapies are available for use in end-of-life care and to enhance the *Golden Room* experience. Some of these healing modalities and their definitions are listed in Table 3.3. Mariano (2010) aptly explains the client benefits of these integrative therapies, as detailed in Exhibit 3.2. Palliative care also affords comfort measures for a person who is feeling poorly. Light touch is important as it signifies caring and love. Some of these additional options and their significance are described in Table 3.4.

TABLE 3.3   Complementary Modalities

Modality	Description
Centering	Focusing one's thoughts and energy within, thereby quieting the mind
Chakra balancing	An Eastern balancing of the energy centers in the body
Craniosacral therapy	Gentle manual pressure on the skull, spine, and membranes returning rhythmic flow to the craniosacral system
Creating intention	Focusing on the purpose of an activity in the mind
Foot and hand reflexology	Relieving pain by stimulating predetermined pressure points on hands and feet
Healing touch	Noninvasive method utilizing the hands to clear, energize, and balance both the human and environmental energy field
Herbology	The use of herbs to ameliorate symptoms

(Continued)

TABLE 3.3   (*Continued*)

Modality	Description
Homeopathy	Treating persons with heavily diluted preparations based on the law of similars
Imagery	A system of visualization helpful in relaxation
Journaling (often by family members)	Private memoir of events, experiences, and reflections
M technique	A simple stroking technique to relieve pain, anxiety, or distress
Massage	Gentle rubbing of both muscle and connective tissue to improve the function of those tissues and encourage relaxation and well-being by easing tension and lessening pain
Meditation	Quiet reflection and contemplation
Prayer	Personal communication with a higher power/God
Reiki	Simple no-touch hands-on visualization practice to recover life energy flow, thereby lessening stress and pain
Relaxation	Refreshment of mind and body through stopping and being
Reminiscence/life review	Putting life in perspective through looking back; finding meaning and value in one's life or that of a loved one
Sense therapies	Using the senses to promote relaxation and peace
Soothing music	Soft music that is calming to the mind
Spiritual reflection	Relaxation of the mind and emotions through focusing on the truths of God
Therapeutic touch	Returning the body energies to balance through the natural healing force, based on the ancient technique "laying on of hands"
Touch	Closing the space between two people; an act of gentle compassion

EXHIBIT 3.2   Benefits of Holistic Integrative Therapies

1. "Holistic therapies build on the body's capabilities and are aimed toward strengthening the body's own defenses and healing abilities so that it can do for itself. Strengthening and healthy defenses offer relief that exceeds symptom management."
2. "Holistic therapies empower clients and families. People are taught about self-care practices, guided in using them, and assisted in exploring obstacles that could stand in the way of doing so."
3. "Most holistic therapies are safer and gentler than conventional therapies. A variety of physical and mental changes, combined with the high volume and nature of medications used in terminal phases of illnesses, carry many risks for dying clients."

From Mariano (2010, p. 52).

Physical touching, which is a human phenomenon, is common to most comfort measures. Significant physical comfort measures that include the sense of touch convey the message "you are not alone" and quietly support the person and the family and assure them of deep respect and dignity as the end of life encroaches. We in America have come to expect touch as an important component in feeling loved and cared for. On the purely physical level, being touched decreases the space between people and not only gives comfort but in the act itself symbolizes "caring." Touch assists many people in uniting with their higher power.

TABLE 3.4   Comfort Measures and Their Significance

Comfort Measures	Significance
Light touch	Love and caring
Gentle massage of legs, arms, and/or back	Soothing
Pain relief	Sympathy and compassion
Positional changes	Consideration
Rocking and holding	Calming and relaxing
Words of comfort and caring	Kindness and consoling

Words of Wisdom

"Caring for families with a member awaiting the end of life creates a situation where the presence of an inevitable death demands that nurses create close relationships with each unique person involved"

From Iranmanesh, Häggström, Axelsson, and Sävenstedt (2009).

FAMILY RITUALS

Family rituals and acts of coming together to be with the dying person are embraced. These include singing, holding hands, speaking remembrances of times past, laughing, being in the moment to support the person, and remembering that the sense of hearing is the last to go so words are heard after the sense of touch is gone.

Often family rituals include the extended family and the bringing in of traditional foods. It becomes a time of "watchful waiting" and a quiet celebration of the life of the honored guest—the dying person. At other times a single person might be present who is quietly dying with the patient, who is the love of that person's life. This individual may have centered his or her life on caring for the patient. Whatever the circumstance, all are welcome to celebrate and are free to express their family rituals in the *Golden Room.*

The dignified, personalized attention offered in the *Golden Room* is based on the understanding that the person dying is the best teacher to show the health care providers what is needed and how the care needs to be given. As a result the care of each person is unique and individualized to bring forth all the aspects of goodness, compassion, peace, dignity, and release.

In the *Golden Room* the caregiver can assist the person to open to the moment several times during the day (Olson & Dossey, 2009). This can be for 10 minutes, or longer or shorter depending on the condition and attention span of the dying person. This is a time for moving within and beginning to feel the gentle peace that passes understanding. This offers comfort in the moment and a gentle guide to go within as the moment of passage approaches. The guided imagery script in Exhibit 3.3 is an example of the type of gentle assistance that is available in the *Golden Room* as one is approaching death.

Yes, there is a place for death with dignity, the *Golden Room*. Very quickly as *Golden Rooms* come to hospitals, nursing homes, and free-standing facilities, you as nurses will experience the breath of relief, the relaxing and letting go that take place for the patients. If you are transferring or discharging the patient to the *Golden Room*, you will likely see the anticipation of release. If you are admitting a patient to the *Golden Room*, you will likely see the response, "Yes, it is time, I'm here." As entry into the delivery room heralds imminent arrival of a newborn, so entry into the *Golden Room* heralds the imminent departure of a loved one. There is an almost palpable feeling of relief, such joy in being surrounded by loving, caring family, friends, and personnel who are assisting in these last days, these last minutes. The struggle is over for everyone, patient and family: No more tubes, no more tests, no more pushing and poking. And with this gentle realization there is a resting, a deep comfort that arises from within. All is well.

Families will also discover that although death can be a bittersweet experience, the loss is cradled in the arms of loving personnel, a gentle ambiance, and a depth of compassion and caring for them as well as the patient. Here they also are treated as honored guests on this journey of a lifetime.

EXHIBIT 3.3   Guided Imagery Script

See within you a gentle light . . . so soft . . . so warm and inviting . . . allow yourself to gently move toward the light . . . no effort here . . . gradually allow yourself to go closer and closer . . . so inviting, so loving . . . gently, so gently begin to feel the light surrounding you . . . caressing you . . . inviting you deeper . . . quietly let go of the room and your surroundings as you go further and further into the light . . . so gentle . . . so loving . . . tenderly release your loved ones, as you go deeper . . . no hurry here, you have plenty of time . . . feel the lightness . . . so loving . . . so inviting . . . everything is being taken care of here . . . you are loved . . . keep moving deeper into the light . . . gently feel yourself becoming the light . . . feel the lightness . . . the radiance . . . the only thing left is the sound of my voice . . . just keep going into the love . . . into the light . . . my voice begins to fade as you move deeper into the light . . . it's okay . . . you are so loved . . . so safe and comfortable . . . don't let anything hold you back . . . you are loved . . . you are remembered . . . keep going . . . keep going . . . into the light.

EXHIBIT 3.4   Research Perspective

It comes as no surprise to nurses when studies validate the preponderance of time that they spend with patients compared to time spent by other health care professionals. One study indicated that in a population of 58 dying patients, attending physicians spent an average of only 3 minutes per day with each patient. House staff visits averaged 9 minutes, while visits by nursing personnel averaged 45 minutes. Even family members visited for an average of only 13 minutes per day. Although study findings indicated that seriously ill patients ended up spending almost 19 hours per day alone, the authors also found that no patients in the hospital received much more attention.

Studies like this give us important data. We learn that dying patients at least receive a comparable amount of attention from health care providers as other patients, but no one gets enough time, and it is nurses who provide the most attention and care.

From Carroll-Johnson (2001).

As nurses we can feel not only the sense of relief that accompanies being admitted to the *Golden Room* but also the deep sense of gratitude for this final dignity in the life of the loved one. Quite possibly what was once the last place that a nurse would want to work, with the old and dying, the *Golden Room* becomes a place nurses are eager to participate in. Here nursing is all about nursing. Here nurses have the time to sit and be with the patient and the family. Here the nurses are expected to be in the room and give the comfort measures they learned so long ago in their beginning education. Here the ideals of nursing become the reality of nursing. Here is the *Golden Room* (Exhibit 3.4).

CRITERIA FOR ADMISSION

The admission criteria for the *Golden Room* are simple and straightforward:

1. The person is within 3–10 days of death.
2. A physician's order to be transferred has been written.
3. The person/family has requested/has been offered the *Golden Room* and has accepted.

4. The person understands that all life-support techniques will be removed before transport, but palliative comfort care will still be given.
5. The person, or the family, has signed the appropriate admission papers.

Golden Room centers can become an expected part of the health care delivery system. Just as there are labor and delivery centers in most acute care and community hospitals, it seems very natural to expect *Golden Room* centers to be developed in hospitals and nursing homes in the future. It is, however, important to note that the *Golden Room* is not for everyone. Many people are blessed with end-of-life care at home. They have supportive and able family members who can be with them during a natural death at home. Many other terminal patients have the added benefit of hospice. Hospice nurses work with the family to administer pain medications, offer palliative care, and help the household members cope with the process. These are the fortunate few. At this point in our evolution there are still countless thousands who at any one time suffer the consequences of a solitary and/or painful death. They are alone, without family or friends. Their prognosis is grim, and other than suppressive medication, little is done about it. *The Golden Room* is a place for a goodness, compassion, peace, dignity, and release that is soon to come.

SUMMARY

Never in the history of our country have we had so many people dying as well as so many who will die soon. We are ill prepared with places to go for our last days when efforts overwhelm those caring for the dying at home or when patients have been in acute care settings and nursing homes.

The Golden Room offers the concept of creating a new place for dying, a place that offers patients death with dignity and the family a place to feel at home as they tend to their loved one. This room offers the patient a place to be a person of dignity and worth, uncluttered with all the physical artificially life-prolonging devices, and to simply experience the comfort of family and loved ones in a supportive atmosphere. *The Golden Room* offers the family the privacy, the time, the opportunity, and the support to come together and laugh and cry. The trained and compassionate staff are able to support, comfort, and love the patient and family while assisting them through this special one-of-a-kind, never-to-be-repeated experience that we call physical death.

REFERENCES

Carroll-Johnson, R. M. (2001). Nursing diagnoses at the end of life. *Nursing Diagnosis, 4*.

Carvalho, W. B., Pedreira, M. L. G., & deAguiar, M. A. L. (2005). Noise level in a pediatric intensive care unit. *Journal of Pediatrics Intensive Care Units, 81*(6), 496–497.

Centers for Disease Control and Prevention/National Center for Health Statistics. (2009). Retrieved April 28, 2010, from http://www.cdc.gov/nchs/FASTATS/deaths.htm

Iranmanesh, S., Häggström, T., Axelsson, K., & Sävenstedt, S. (2009). Swedish nurses' experiences of caring for dying people: A holistic approach. *Holistic Nursing Practice, 23*(4), 243–252.

Mariano, C. (2010). Holistic integrative therapies in palliative care. In M. Matzo & D. Sherman (Eds.), *Palliative care nursing* (p. 52). New York: Springer Publishing Company.

Morris, D. L. (2009). Music therapy. In B. M. Dossey & L. Keegan, *Holistic nursing: A handbook for practice* (5th ed.). Sudbury, MA: Jones & Bartlett, 327–336.

Mularski, R. A., Puntillo, K., Varkey, B., Erstad, B. L., Grap, M. J., Gilbert, H. C., et al. (2009). Pain management within the palliative and end-of-life care experience in the ICU. *Chest, 135*(5), 1360–1369.

Olson, M., & Dossey, B. M. (2009). Dying in peace. In B. M. Dossey & L. Keegan, *Holistic nursing: A handbook for practice* (5th ed., p. 339). Sudbury, MA: Jones & Bartlett.

O'Mahony, S., McHenry, J., Blank, A. E., Snow, D., Karakas, S. E., Santoro, G., et al. (2010). Preliminary report of the integration of a palliative care team into an intensive care unit. *Palliative Medicine, 24*(2), 154–165.

4 End-of-Life Issues

Health is not only to be well, but to use well every power we have.
—Florence Nightingale, 1893

*B*ERNARD'S STORY *Bernard was a retired forest ranger with a wife, four grown children, and three grandchildren. Three months prior to his 74th birthday he began to have persistent stomach pains that were unrelieved by his longtime use of antacids and laxatives. Although he began to take Tylenol, there was no relief, so reluctantly after his birthday he made an appointment to see his family physician.*

Three months later at his appointment he was having dark, tarry stools and becoming very constipated; laxatives were no longer helpful. A physical exam revealed a distended abdomen with rigidity and rebound tenderness. Bernard was immediately hospitalized for a colonoscopy and multiple lab tests, which revealed a large mass in the lower colon, intersusception, and a constriction in the rectal vault. He was advised that immediate surgery was necessary to save his life, with a probable permanent colostomy.

Bernard, shaking, called his wife and shared his bad news. Helen immediately called the children and headed for the hospital, which was over an hour away. She remembered to bring his living will and power of attorney from the health document file. When Helen reached the hospital, quite shaken and white, she found Bernard on the medical-surgical floor. She was unprepared for what she saw. Her strong, virile husband was curled on his side in bed with an IV and a Foley catheter, and he was heavily sedated. Groggily Bernard told her that the gastroenterology consult had recommended immediate surgery and he had consented. The preoperative electrocardiogram revealed a slight heart murmur and prehypertension. He was considered high risk for surgery. A second and third consult concurred that the surgery should be attempted given the grave prognosis. Things were moving very fast, yet Helen remembered to give the nurse Bernard's living will and power of attorney.

Bernard was whisked to surgery, and Helen left to collect herself in the surgery waiting room. The children arrived and sat with their mother for what seemed like an eternity. In the late evening the surgeon talked with them, saying that Bernard had survived the surgery with a colostomy; both the mass and the intersusception had been removed, but the rectal vault stricture was unfixable. Bernard was weak from blood loss and "heart irregularities."

When Helen finally saw her husband he was ashen and would not look at her nor respond to her but pulled away from her touch. Helen and her children took turns sitting with Bernard as permitted in the intensive care unit (ICU). He refused to acknowledge them. In 24 hours his temperature became elevated and his abdominal dressing had increasing seepage. Lab tests including blood gases determined that Bernard had an infection. Massive antibiotics were started along with nasal oxygen as his breathing was becoming labored and intense. More consults and laboratory tests were ordered as Bernard continued to go downhill. It was a long night for Bernard's family. As the sun rose the next morning, Bernard slipped into unconsciousness only to open his eyes briefly and look at his wife; he then passed away with the buzz of machines and respirators in the background.

REFLECTIONS ON ISSUES OF CONCERN

1. If death is a natural part of the life cycle, when is this natural part "allowed" to happen?
2. How do we dignify the unexpected dying and death of a middle-aged person when the focus is on treating and keeping him or her alive? At what point is enough enough?
3. How do we begin to discuss the end of life and become aware of this natural process?
4. How comfortable are you with talking about your mortality or with your parents about their mortality?
5. What are the criteria for medical futility?
6. What are the criteria for death with dignity?
7. Is the acute care setting the best place to say goodbye? Or is there a better place, such as the *Golden Room*?

DEATH: A NATURAL PART OF THE LIFE CYCLE

As a culture and as a society we have nicely prepared for entry into life. Birthing centers are in place in most hospitals. Lamaze classes and childbirth-preparation books proliferate. What just a couple of generations ago used to be a private and oftentimes-frightening phenomenon, both for the patient and the family, has evolved to become an event that is openly and easily talked about. Preparation for and acceptance of childbirth as natural and good are well established.

Despite the wonderful advances made in the past couple of decades, the end of life is an area still in need of development and considerable change. The fact is that we have as many people dying as being born, yet a stigma against openly talking about death and dying remains. For the most part death is discussed privately, and seldom and generally not at all until the time for a family member's departure grows near and then mainly in hushed, hurried voices.

END-OF-LIFE AWARENESS

In 2002, members of the Healthy Aging Team of the Centers for Disease Control (CDC) collaborated with colleagues from the Division of Cancer Prevention and Control and the Association of State and Territorial Chronic Disease Directors, now known as the National Association for Chronic Disease Directors (NACDD), to develop public health priorities for end-of-life issues. This work involved 200 key public health stakeholders and resulted in 103 short-, intermediate-, and long-term priorities.

The top five initial priorities were

1. Identifying a point of contact for end-of-life issues in state health departments
2. Collecting and analyzing data about the end of life
3. Incorporating end-of-life principles into state comprehensive cancer control plans
4. Educating the public about hospice and palliative care
5. Educating the public about the importance of advance directives and health care proxies (CDC, n.d.).

These top five initial priorities form the framework for many current projects that focus on end-of-life issues. None of these priorities speaks to shifting our consciousness about dying and death, nor do they speak to the need for special attention to the quality of life while dying.

END-OF-LIFE ISSUES

Effective public health strategies and medical treatment advances have resulted in a 30-year increase in life expectancy in the last 100 years. As people live longer, their expectations about quality of life throughout the life span, including at its very end, are increasing. The fact is that death itself is ultimately not preventable, and most people will die as a result of chronic disease (CDC, n.d.).

The end of life is associated with a substantial burden of suffering among many dying individuals as well as health and financial consequences that extend to family members and society. The data indicate that as many as 50% of dying persons with cancer or other chronic illnesses experience unrelieved symptoms during their final days. Furthermore, recent studies demonstrate an increased likelihood of depressive symptoms and mortality among caregivers of terminally ill patients. Because most deaths occur in hospitals, end-of-life care has been recognized as an important clinical issue needing improvement.

Much of the suffering that may accompany terminal illness is amenable to interventions that are often not accessible to everyone. For instance, studies point to disparities in hospice use, particularly among patients with certain types of cancer, such as prostate cancer. It is uncertain whether these disparities are due to lack of awareness regarding the options for end-of-life care or to differences in perspectives regarding the end of life (CDC, n.d.).

Medical Futility

Medical futility is a concept commonly used to describe medical therapy that has no known or anticipated immediate- or long-term benefit for a patient. This is especially true for end-of-life issues. The concept of futility has existed since the time of Hippocrates and has become the predominant dilemma for many end-of-life situations. Nurses grapple with issues of medical futility in their daily practice and use the concept when they are talking with patients and families who are in a quandary about their loved one's care (Whitmer, Hurst, Prins, Shepard, & McVey,

2009). This and other ethical issues are discussed in Chapter 6. Exhibit 4.1 offers food for thought about medical futility.

Withholding and Withdrawing Care

There is definite crossover between end-of-life issues and the ethics of end-of-life care. Certainly, withholding and/or withdrawal of care is one of the issues that relate to both topics. Actually, the most difficult decisions about withholding treatments often relate to some of the simpler, noninvasive therapies, such as use of antibiotics, and those that are symbolically linked to caring and nurturing, such as providing food and fluids (Schwartz & Tarzian, 2010). In general, it is easier to withhold a treatment (not begin it) than to withdraw it. For example, when people take the time to prepare an advance directive (see Chapter 2) they consider all the options and determine what would actually be best for them in the long run. In advance they think through and get a pretty good idea of whether they really want such treatments as a feeding tube, respiratory intubation, experimental surgery, extra radiation, and chemotherapy, for example. Learning about and weighing the pros and cons of each life-prolonging therapy increases the knowledge of the individual making end-of-life care decisions. Again, not starting a therapy is easier than withdrawing it once established.

EXHIBIT 4.1 Point of View

Samantha Girard is either being saved by medical technology or being prevented from dying a natural death. You decide.

Samantha is 71 years old, a widow living alone with multiple chronic ailments and suffering from the complications of abdominal surgery and a hospital-acquired infection. She has been unconscious in the intensive care unit for almost a week. The cost range is $5,000 to $10,000 a day to maintain someone in the intensive care unit. Some patients remain here for weeks or even months. Samantha has given up the will to live and refuses food. Her daughter calls from out of state every few days to inquire about her mother's condition. What do you recommend? If *Golden Rooms* were available in your hospital, would you and your team consider transfer? When do we decide that a situation is medically futile? Should quality of life be a factor in decision making?

Adapted from CBS News (2009).

Withdrawal of care becomes more complicated. For example, artificial feeding via feeding tubes or intravenous lines becomes a fixed, somewhat invasive procedure. This distinguishes the treatment as artificial in contrast to oral intake of food and water, which is natural. Some clinicians view withdrawal of life support or life-prolonging treatments as passive euthanasia while others think of it as allowing the natural process to unfold, letting one die. There is no clear ethical or moral consensus on many of these issues (Schwartz & Tarzian, 2010). However, a moral and legal consensus concludes that artificial nutrition and hydration may be refused or withdrawn on the same grounds as any other medical intervention. Most of these life-prolonging interventions are weighed and decided on the estimation of the expected benefit or burden to the patient (Beauchamp & Childress, 2008).

THE RIGHT PLACE TO SAY GOOD-BYE

Is there a right place or a wrong place to say good-bye? When an individual is terminal, then there may be a correct answer. Is it, for example, in the ICU? Nurses who work there and do not know of or have any other options speak of their plight when they say no death is easy, but they hope to assist their patients to die peacefully, with their loved ones surrounding them, comforted by each other's presence, and knowing that the right decision has been made. Where and how people die is a significant issue. Exhibit 4.2 highlights one research study in this area.

Quite telling in Exhibit 4.2 is the nurses' attempt to provide dignified end-of-life care and give the relatives softer memories of a peaceful death at the end to somehow offset the suffering and multiple tests and machines in the high-technology ICU. And yet nurses' end-of-life care was focused primarily around their interaction with the family. Interestingly, the persons dying alone, while thought to be heartbreaking, left a much lesser memory for the nurses. While in some ways this is understandable, these persons dying alone must be considered. No one should have to die alone. Where is the dignity? Where is the compassion? Where is the nurse and the caring associated with nursing?

Not knowing of any alternative, many ICU nurses hope for a comfortable place for the patient and his/her loved ones and the nursing staff and physicians to say goodbye. Again, not knowing options, these nurses try to make the ICU a comfortable place for the dying patients and their loved ones and by doing so also make the patients' deaths comfortable for themselves (Millner, Paskiewicz, & Kautz, 2009). Hence,

EXHIBIT 4.2   Research Perspective

One recent study in Sweden explored nurses' experiences and perceptions of caring for dying patients in an ICU, with a focus on unaccompanied patients, the proximity of family members, and environmental aspects. Interviews were conducted with nine experienced ICU nurses using a qualitative descriptive approach. The analysis resulted in a main category, doing one's utmost, described by four generic categories and 15 subcategories, comprising a common vision of the patients' last hours and dying process. This description was dominated by the nurses' endeavor to provide dignified end-of-life care and, when relatives were present, to give them an enduring memory of their loved one's death as a calm and dignified event despite his or her previous suffering and death in a high-technological environment. Nurses' end-of-life care was mainly described as their relationship and interaction with the dying patients' relatives, while patients who died alone were considered tragic but left a lesser impression in the nurses' memory.

From Fridh, De Gendt, and Bergbom (2009).

Words of Wisdom

"Critical care nurses are often faced with working with families during the end-of-life care of a loved one. Often there is indecisiveness in family members of critically ill patients when faced with making these difficult decisions."

From Browning (2009, p. 18).

the issue here is, are we as professionals and as a society ready to let go of having patients come to their end in ICUs? The time has come to create a new place for death with dignity, *Golden Rooms*.

TRENDS IN OTHER CULTURES

When we look at different continents and the range of countries and cultures on each, it is fascinating to compare and contrast the similarities and differences in end-of-life issues and practices between each.

Europe

On the European continent, the Netherlands and Belgium have the most liberal end-of-life policies. Euthanasia, the premeditated use of a terminal dose of hypnotics, is legal in both countries. Researchers recently studied and compared official documents relating to the Belgian and the Dutch NCE-procedures (Notifying, controlling, and evaluating) for euthanasia. In both countries, physicians are required to notify a review committee of their cases, stimulating them to safeguard the quality of their euthanasia practice and making societal control over the practice of euthanasia possible. The main differences between them are that the Dutch notification and control procedures are more elaborate and transparent than the Belgian ones. The Belgian procedures are primarily anonymous, whereas the Dutch ones are not. Societal evaluation is made in both countries through the committees' summary reports to the parliament. The researchers believe that the transparent procedures practiced by the Dutch may better facilitate societal control. Informing physicians about the law and the due care requirements for euthanasia and providing systematic feedback about their medical actions are both pivotal to achieving efficient societal control and engendering the level of care needed when performing such far-reaching medical acts (Smets et al., 2009).

Recently, continuous deep sedation is becoming more common than euthanasia in the Netherlands for terminally ill patients who are nearing death. Deep sedation is often used when other methods of controlling pain or discomfort fail. The technique can be used intermittently or continuously until death occurs. The level of sedation can vary from a lowered state of consciousness to unconsciousness. Patients are often kept in deep sedation for several days before they die. The rise in the use of continuous deep sedation for patients nearing death in the Netherlands suggests that this practice is increasingly considered part of regular medical practice (Reinberg, 2008).

Switzerland also has a liberal right-to-die policy. The nonphysician volunteers of Exit, the largest right-to-die organization in Switzerland, play an important role in assisted suicide. They conduct assessments and deliver lethal medications for a member to self-administer (Bosshard, Ulrich, Ziegler, & Bär, 2008).

About half of the persons who die in developed countries are very old (80 years of age or older), and this proportion is still rising. The odd thing is, however, that end-of-life decision making is less common for very old than for younger patients. A recent Belgian study found that physicians seem to have a more reluctant attitude toward the use of lethal drugs, terminal sedation, and participation in decision making when dealing with very old patients. The study therefore recommends that advance care planning should increase the involvement of very old competent and noncompetent patients in end-of-life decision making (De Gendt, Bilsen, Mortier, Vander Stichele, & Deliens, 2008).

Australia

On the Australian continent there has been much debate regarding the double effect of sedatives and analgesics administered at the end of life and the possibility that health professionals using these drugs are performing "slow euthanasia." On the one hand, analgesics and sedatives can do much to relieve suffering in the terminally ill. On the other hand, they can hasten death. According to a standard view, the administration of analgesics and sedatives amounts to euthanasia when the drugs are given with an intention to hasten death. Researchers found a striking ambiguity and uncertainty regarding intentions among the doctors they interviewed. Some were explicit in describing a gray area between palliation and euthanasia, or a continuum between the two. Not one of the respondents was consistent in distinguishing between a foreseen death and an intended death. A major theme was that slow euthanasia may be more psychologically acceptable to doctors than active voluntary euthanasia by bolus injection, partly because the former would usually result in only a small loss of time for patients already very close to death but also because of the desirable ambiguities surrounding causation and intention when an infusion of analgesics and sedatives is used. Empirical and philosophical implications of this double effect must continue to be explored (Douglas, Kerridge, & Ankeny, 2008).

Mexico

Mexico is a large country with a growing population. A group of researchers sought information on what Mexicans think of physician-assisted death. They sampled 2,097 individuals from several specialties employed by a Mexican government health system, distributed throughout the country. Approximately 40% supported physicians helping terminally ill patients who request to die because of intolerable suffering caused by incurable diseases, whereas 44% said no, and the rest were undecided. This was statistically different from the answers to the scenario in which the relatives of a patient in a persistent vegetative state ask their physician to help him or her die, where 48% of respondents said yes, and 35% said no. The main reasons to say yes in both scenarios were respect for patients' or families' autonomy and avoidance of suffering, whereas those opposed cited other ethical and mainly religious considerations. The variable associated with the highest probability of approving of both scenarios was legal in nature, whereas strong religious beliefs were against accepting physicianassisted death. The group was evenly divided, with approximately 40% each for and against the idea of helping a patient die and approximately 20% undecided (Lisker, Alvarez Del Rio, Villa, & Carnevale, 2008).

China

China has set up an association to address end-of-life care for one of the world's largest aging populations. The Chinese Association for Life Care acts as a nationwide regulatory organization in the field of end-of-life care. The association, composed of medical workers, legal workers, and volunteers, engages in the development of end-of-life care, palliative care, gerontology research, and health care for the elderly. The mission is to regulate services across the nation, organizing academic communication and domestic and international exchanges to improve the quality of care in China.

"Life care" means the provision of services for elderly people, especially dying people, and allowing them to die with dignity. China has three forms of life-care services: a small number of end-of-life care hospitals, about 200 end-of-life wards in medical institutions, and hospices. There are 143 million people over the age of 60 in China, accounting for 11% of the population (Xunhua, 2006).

Cultures vary in their beliefs regarding death and dying as reflected in their laws and practices. One thing is apparent: Each is searching for ways to bring dignity to death and to assist both the person and the family in this time of transition. *The Golden Room* is certainly another option for them to consider. As the United States embraces and implements *Golden Rooms*, they can easily and naturally spread to other countries.

PLANNING FOR THE END OF LIFE

Family members are often asked to make decisions on behalf of a loved one who is seriously ill without having a complete understanding of his or her preferences. To avoid this situation, older adults need to discuss their end-of-life wishes with family members and health care providers well before the onset of a serious illness, and they should designate a surrogate decision maker for health care.

EXHIBIT 4.3   Basic Communication Skills to Foster Meaningful Conversations

- Asking open-ended questions
- Asking for validation
- Asking "how" or "what" questions
- Making reflective statements
- Asking clarifying questions
- Repeating in question form

Having these conversations is the best way to protect one's independence in myriad unpredictable situations. However, many people find it difficult to begin a discussion about end-of-life issues. Fortunately, several resources are available to help foster meaningful conversations and practical planning for end-of-life care. Exhibit 4.3 details some of those basic communication skills.

On closer scrutiny, the basic communication skills may seem vaguely familiar, and in fact these were learned in most nurses' initial education. These skills certainly can get one started and begin to open the door. However, they are foundational and are only the tip of the iceberg for moving into a conversation about death and dying.

BEGINNING A CONVERSATION
ABOUT DEATH AND DYING

As nurses our focus is to assist patients to look at themselves and work through their feelings about death and dying so they can become more comfortable both in the process and in talking about death with their family and friends. There is one caveat here: The success of these communications goes only as far as the nurse is comfortable with his or her own feelings about death and dying. This inner work is imperative for nurses, families, and, yes, the dying person.

Often we think that we are comfortable with our own death only to discover that as we share this with other people their responses are often surprising. Often we can feel their hesitation to think about, much less talk about, our or their death and dying. The out-of-sight, out-of-mind comfortable discomfort becomes apparent. It is easy to talk about a living will, advance directives, and a power of attorney yet never talk about how we are feeling or what we want our loved ones to know about our life, our preferences, and our discoveries in our life.

The easiest way to begin to become comfortable with talking about our death or a loved one's death and dying is to start with a simple, "I want to share with you about something that is important to me and I hope that we can get beyond our uncomfortableness and simply share from our hearts." Whatever the words are, however they come out, the most important part is to speak from an open, loving heart. This and other advanced skills to foster meaningful conversations about the end of life are outlined in Exhibit 4.4. Exhibit 4.5 portrays one study of a technique to help focus a meaningful conversation.

EXHIBIT 4.4   Advanced Skills to Foster Meaningful Conversations about the End of Life

- Speak from an open heart
- Be in this moment
- Acknowledge your feelings to yourself
- Allow yourself to feel the feelings
- Observe the inner shifting in your feelings as you listen and talk

EXHIBIT 4.5   Research Perspective

A "Go Wish" card game was designed to allow patients to consider the importance of common issues at the end of life in a nonconfrontational setting. By sorting through their values in private, patients may be better able to have a focused conversation about end-of-life care. Investigators sought to evaluate the feasibility of using the Go Wish card game with seriously ill patients in the hospital. Of the 133 subjects, the value selected as the highest in importance by the most subjects was to be pain free. Other highly ranked values concerned spirituality, maintaining a sense of self, symptom management, and establishing a strong relationship with health care professionals. Average time to review the patients' ranked list after the patients sorted their values in private was 21.8 minutes (range: 6–45 minutes). These results suggest that it is feasible to use the Go Wish card game to obtain an accurate portrayal of a patient's care goals in a time-efficient manner.

From Lankarani-Fard et al. (2010).

Although these advanced skills appear to be simple and straightforward, they require much practice and honest self-reflection, and they lead to huge growth in awareness and the ability to work with patients of all backgrounds and situations. As nurses become more aware of their "inner terrain," of their own feelings around death and dying, these advanced skills begin to emerge and strengthen naturally.

How fortunate it is when the person dying is comfortable with himself or herself and can help lead the way. How fortunate it is when the family learns to speak from their hearts, even if it is not easy or fun; this deep sharing brings such great rewards for all involved. How fortunate it is when the nurses are comfortable with their own mortality. Each time death is talked about it becomes easier. For the dying person, knowing that your family is there to help walk through this last physical journey lends to a dignified death. Knowing that as family you can speak openly to the dying person from your heart is healing. Knowing that there are caregivers that are specially trained to assist us is comforting. We are all strong, far stronger than we know, and we discover that inner core of strength as we speak and listen from our hearts.

In the *Golden Room* there is time to share, time to be, time to hold, time to love, and time to say good-bye, with memories to cherish, as dignity and love become the passwords.

SUMMARY

Advance care proxies, living wills, education of the public, and the incorporation of end-of-life statements at the state level—all these and others are an enormous start in setting the foundational materials in place for end-of-life care. These are already in progress and in various states of completion. The fact remains that most deaths occur within the hospital, and the care of the dying remains a huge clinical issue that not only needs to be not only improved but also changed. It begs the question to speak of medical futility and do nothing to change what is. It begs the question to argue about withholding and withdrawing care for the dying person and do nothing to change what is. We tend to get caught up in mental arguments while people are suffering. Is it not time to become proactive rather than reactive? The ambulance at the bottom of the mountain pales in comparison to fixing the road at the top. It is time to fix the road at the top of the mountain.

This book is a proactive stance for death with dignity. Unless the dying person and his or her family can talk openly and with ease about these and other concerns, the foundation will not be adequately utilized.

Unless health care professionals become comfortable with death and dying as a natural part of the life cycle and reflect that in their practice, the foundation cannot be adequately utilized. Unless death and dying become an easier part of the general discussion among family and friends, the foundation cannot be adequately utilized. Unless the existing foundation is built on through adding the means to give everyone the opportunity for death with dignity, the foundation cannot be adequately utilized.

A huge expansion of consciousness around death and dying is required on all levels to adequately utilize and expand the structures that are being put in place at the national and state levels. Let us begin this massive adjustment within the health care community. Let us become proactive and lead the way. *The Golden Room* is an immense initiative whose time has come.

REFERENCES

Beauchamp, T., & Childress, J. (2008). *Principles of biomedical ethics* (6th ed.). New York: Oxford University Press.

Bosshard, G., Ulrich, E., Ziegler, S. J., & Bär, W. (2008). Assessment of requests for assisted suicide by a Swiss right-to-die society. *Death Studies, 32*(7), 646–657.

Browning, A. M. (2009). Empowering family members in end-of-life care decision making in the intensive care unit. *Dimensions in Critical Care Nursing, 28*(1), 18–23.

CBS News. (2009, November 23). *The cost of dying.* Retrieved May 3, 2010, from http://www.wkrg.com/financial/article/the_cost_of_dying/541220/Nov-23-2009_12-07-pm/

Centers for Disease Control and Prevention. *The State of Aging and Health in America.* (2007). Whitehouse Station, NJ: The Merck Company Foundation. Retrieved May 3, 2010, from www.cdc.gov/Aging/saha.htm

Centers for Disease Control and Prevention. (n.d.) "Aging." Retrieved May 3, 2010, from http://www.cdc.gov/Aging/EOL.htm

De Gendt, C., Bilsen, J., Mortier, F., Vander Stichele, R., & Deliens, L. (2008). End-of-life decision-making and terminal sedation among very old patients. *Gerontology, 55*(1), 99–105.

Douglas, C., Kerridge, I., & Ankeny, R. (2008, August). Managing intentions: The end-of-life administration of analgesics and sedatives, and the possibility of slow euthanasia. *Bioethics, 22*(7), 388–396.

Fridh, I., De Gendt, C., & Berghom, I. (2009). Doing one's utmost: Nurses' descriptions of caring for dying patients in an intensive care environment. *Intensive Critical Care Nursing, 25*(5), 233–241.

Lankarani-Fard, A., Knapp, H., Lorenz, K. A., Golden, J. F., Taylor, A., Feld, J. E., et al. (2010). Feasibility of discussing end-of-life care goals with inpatients using a structured, conversational approach: The Go Wish card game. *Journal of Pain Symptom Management, 39*(4), 637–643.

Lisker, R., Alvarez Del Rio, A., Villa, A. R., & Carnevale, A. (2008). Physician-assisted death: Opinions of a sample of Mexican physicians. *Archives of Medical Research, 39*(4), 452–458.

Millner, P., Paskiewicz, S. T., & Kautz, D. (2009). A comfortable place to say goodbye. *Dimensions of Critical Care Nursing, 28*(1), 13–17.

Reinberg, S. (2008, March 21). Deep sedation becoming more common for dying patients in Holland. *U.S. News and World Report.* Retrieved May 3, 2010, from http://health.usnews.com/usnews/health/healthday/080321/deep-sedation-becoming-more-common-for-dying-patients-in-holland.htm

Schwartz, K. S., & Tarzian, A. T. (2010). Ethical aspects of palliative care. In M. Matzo & D. W. Sherman (Eds.), *Palliative care nursing.* New York: Springer Publishing Company, 119–141.

Smets, T., Bilsen, J., Cohen, J., Rurup, M. L., De Keyser, E., & Deliens, L. (2009). The medical practice of euthanasia in Belgium and the Netherlands: Legal notification, control and evaluation procedures. *Health Policy, 90*(2–3), 181.

Whitmer, M., Hurst, S., Prins, M., Shepard, K., & McVey, D. (2009). Medical futility: A paradigm as old as Hippocrates. *Dimensions of Critical Care Nursing, 28*(2), 67–71.

Xunhua. (2006, April 17). China gears up to improve end-of-life care. *China Daily.com.* Retrieved May 3, 2010, from http://www.chinadaily.com.cn/china/2006-04/17/content_569087.htm

5 End-of-Life Costs of Care

Doctors often order unnecessary diagnostic tests, procedures and therapies to cover their butts in case of a legal dispute.
—Arthur Caplan, PhD, Director, Center for Bioethics, University of Pennsylvania

JACOB'S STORY   Jacob was a 77-year-old retired auto worker who had been experiencing progressive dementia and Parkinson's symptoms for the past two years. His work provided a health plan for retirement that covered anything not covered by Medicare, but not the over $40,000 his wife, Elizabeth, spent on home health care the previous year. Because of his desire to remain in the home, Elizabeth and their five children asked the physician to write an order for hospice home care and the physician agreed. One morning while transferring Jacob from the transport chair to the bed the caregiver shouted, "Call 911." In a moment of terror, forgetting the hospice plan to not intervene in the dying process, Jacob's wife immediately called the paramedics. Jacob was transported to the hospital via ambulance. The family suspected a stroke or possibly a seizure but received no definitive diagnosis.

In the hospital Jacob's color remained ashen, and his pulse weak and slow. Jacob would shake his head when offered food and stopped talking. Although he passed the swallow test his wife was advised to have a peg tube inserted or do nothing. Jacob had a living will that stated that he did not want an artificial feeding tube. His wife had power of attorney for his health care decisions. Upon consulting the children and knowing nothing about the physical dying process, Elizabeth agreed to the peg tube.

After three weeks of repeated diagnostic tests, at a total cost of $38,996.50, Jacob's status continued to deteriorate, and the physician ordered a transfer to a long-term care facility. The original home hospice agency would not take him back since the family had failed in following the agreed plan of care for a natural death without intervention. The family was unable to locate another hospice, and Jacob was finally transferred to a nursing home. Jacob developed a urinary tract infection *and pneumonia. His decline continued despite the medications and treatments. As it became evident that Jacob was dying, the family implored the physician to discharge Jacob to die at home, which had been Jacob's original intent. The physician agreed and wrote the order for in-home hospice care. Frustration mounted as the error made in calling 911 became more evident. Finally the family found another in-home hospice that would accept Jacob.*

Jacob was discharged to return home after two weeks in the nursing home and four weeks in care facilities. He now had pneumonia, a urinary tract infection, excoriated buttocks, and the peg tube. Jacob's daughters and three brothers came home to help care for Jacob through reminiscing, praying, reading Scripture, and watching his favorite movies. Once at home, Jacob refused nutrition through the peg tube and accepted only morphine by mouth. Each day he declined dramatically.

Eleven days after he returned home Jacob died peacefully at home after countless thousands of dollars had been spent on the hospital, nursing home, and out-of-pocket expenses.

REFLECTIONS ON ISSUES OF CONCERN

1. How do families without insurance or a supplemental insurance policy pay for end-of-life care without wiping out their entire savings or going bankrupt?
2. Who is responsible for the error in calling 911? Is it the caretaker trained to work with hospice and those dying, or is it the wife, who is terrified and unprepared for the sudden change in health and what might be happening?
3. As the cost of end-of-life care soars and needless testing and procedures are done, would one solution be rationing health care? Who would make this decision? What could be the criteria?
4. Do the laws about Medicare need to be changed because of the costs of end-of-life care? Medicare currently cannot deny care on the basis of its cost.
5. The cost of end-of-life care varies greatly across the country. What can be done to equalize this? Is cost of care related to quality of care?
6. Do the costs of end-of-life care need to be explained to the family as part of the decision-making process?

7. Patients without insurance tend to use more resources available to them through social services. Can social services also assist people with insurance to decrease the amount of their copay?

8. Is there any assistance for the out-of-pocket expenses (such as travel and lodging expenses, such as food and taxis) that seem to go unnoticed and unstudied but can end up being very expensive?

9. Many hospices charge for their services. Is this acceptable? What determines their decision to charge or not?

10. End-of-life costs usually increase in the last year of life, with the last 2–4 weeks being the most expensive. What are realistic solutions to these huge end-of-life costs?

Could the *Golden Room* be a solution? With the graying of America, end-of-life care is increasing exponentially and will continue to do so in the decades to come (McCrone, 2009). Serious consideration of the costs of end-of-life care is just beginning. The cost toll detailed in this chapter is in dollars. Not covered here are the overwhelming emotional, psychological, and spiritual end-of-life costs borne by both the patients and their families.

In order to enhance end-of-life care planning, policymakers and decision makers must justify dollar costs (Fassbender, Fainsinger, Carson, & Finegan, 2009). Insurance companies and hospitals alike are reluctant to release information specific to the costs of the last 2 to 4 weeks of life. As a result these expenses have to be determined and examined tangentially and circumspectly.

HOW MUCH DOES DYING COST?

Every medical study ever conducted has concluded that 100% of Americans will eventually die. This comes as no great surprise, but the amount of money being spent at the very end of people's lives will likely be enormous (CBS News, 2009). One in every seven dollars spent on health care is spent during the last 6 months of life. Most Americans say every person deserves life-prolonging care. But is it worth it? Further, can we afford it? Twenty-eight percent of the Medicare budget goes to reimburse people over age 65 in their last year of life. The vast majority is spent in the last 30 days. That sum is about $30 billion. That amount could cover about two-thirds of the cost of providing health care for the 37 million uninsured Americans. About 70% of all who die annually are elderly.

And as the average age of Americans rises (currently 12.5% are over age 65), the cost of care will rise dramatically. The ever-increasing use of new diagnostic and life-prolonging technologies adds more costs. The issue creates a dilemma for all, morally and financially. It seems logical that the most care should be given to those who have a chance to recover (Moody, n.d.)

HOW DID WE GET HERE AND WHERE ARE WE GOING?

Relevant data can be gleaned from looking at the care given in the place where the person died. The Center for Gerontology and Health Care Research, Brown Medical School, Providence, Rhode Island, found that over the past century, nursing homes and hospitals increasingly have become the site of death. However, no national studies had examined the adequacy or quality of end-of-life care in institutional settings compared with deaths at home (Talmor, Shapiro, Greenberg, Stone, & Neumann, 2006). As a result the center set out to evaluate the U.S. experience with dying at home and in institutional settings. The center used a family member or knowledgeable informant mortality follow-back survey representing 1,578 decedents to estimate end-of-life care outcomes for 1.97 million deaths from chronic illness in the United States in 2000. Informants were asked about the patient's experience at the last place of care at which the patient spent more than 48 hours (Talmor et al., 2006). Among the results the following are most pertinent for us:

- For 1,059 of 1,578 decedents (67.1%), the last place of care was an institution.
- Of 519 (32.9%) patients dying at home represented by this sample, 198 (38.2%) did not receive nursing services, 65 (12.5%) had home nursing services, and 256 (49.3%) had home hospice services.
- About one-quarter of all patients with pain or dyspnea did not receive adequate treatment, and one-quarter reported concerns with physician communication.
- More than one-third of respondents cared for by a home health agency, nursing home, or hospital reported insufficient emotional support for the patient and/or one or more concerns with family emotional support, compared with about one-fifth of those receiving home hospice services.
- Nursing home residents were less likely than those cared for in a hospital or by home hospice services to have always been

treated with respect at the end of life (68.2% vs. 79.6% and 96.2%, respectively).

- Family members of patients receiving hospice services were more satisfied with overall quality of care: 70.7% rated care as excellent compared with less than 50% of those whose family member had died in an institutional setting or while receiving home health services.

This study concludes that many people dying in institutions have unmet needs for symptom amelioration, physician communication, emotional support, and respectful treatment. Family members of decedents who received care at home with hospice services were more likely to report a favorable dying experience (Talmor et al., 2006). It is evident from this investigation that the majority of patients (67.1%) die in the hospital in pain and in need of both emotional support and respect. This could be dramatically changed with *Golden Room* suites available in hospitals and nursing homes in addition to freestanding centers in the community (Exhibit 5.1).

EXHIBIT 5.1   Research Perspective

Concern regarding wide variations in spending and intensive care unit use for patients at the end of life (EOL) hinges on the assumption that such treatment offers little or no survival benefit. One study explored the relationship between hospital "end-of-life" treatment intensity and postadmission survival. A retrospective cohort analysis of 1,021,909 patients 65 years old or older, incurring 2,216,815 admissions in 169 Pennsylvania acute care hospitals, was conducted. Researchers used a measure of EOL treatment intensity (a summed index of standardized intensive care unit and life-sustaining treatment use among patients with a high predicted probability of dying [PPD] at admission) and 30- and 180-day postadmission mortality. The results found that there was a nonlinear negative relationship between hospital EOL treatment intensity and 30-day mortality among all admissions, although patients with a higher PPD derived the greatest benefit. **Researchers concluded that admission to hospitals that provide higher EOL treatment intensity is associated with only small gains in postadmission survival.**

From Barnato et al. (2010).

TYPES OF INSURANCE PLANS

Medicare

About one-quarter of Medicare outlays are for the last year of life, a fact that has not changed in the last 20 years (Buntin & Huskamp, 2002). Right now most of the uncontrolled growth in U.S. federal spending and the deficit comes from Medicare. Almost one-third of the money spent by Medicare, about $66.8 billion, goes to chronically ill patients in the last 2 years of life (Emanuel, 1996). Studies have documented poor quality of care, dissatisfaction with care, and limitations in the coverage of end-of-life care for Medicare beneficiaries. However, critical gaps in our knowledge about how to design a better end-of-life care system for Medicare beneficiaries remain (Stevenson & Bramson, 2009).

By law, Medicare cannot reject any treatment based on cost. It will pay $55,000 for patients with advanced breast cancer to receive the chemotherapy drug Avastin, even though it extends life only by an average of a month and a half; it will pay $40,000 for a 93-year-old man with terminal cancer to get a surgically implanted defibrillator if he happens to have heart problems too (CBS News, 2009).

In 2008, Medicare paid $50 billion just for doctor and hospital bills during the last 2 months of patients' lives. That sum is more than the budget of the Department of Homeland Security or the Department of Education. And it has been estimated that 20% to 30% of these medical expenditures may have had no meaningful impact on quality of life, while longevity is only slightly prolonged. Most of the bills are paid for by the federal government with few or no questions asked. It seems unbelievable that as a society we have not adequately addressed these issues of end-of-life care costs (CBS News, 2009).

A researcher at the Dartmouth Institute for Health Policy completed a detailed analysis of Medicare records for patients in the last 2 years of their lives. He found it was more efficient for doctors to manage seriously ill patients in a hospital situation. In addition, there are other incentives that affect the cost and the care patients receive. Among these are the fact that most doctors are paid based on the number of patients they see, and most hospitals are paid for the number of patients they admit.

As the system works now the easiest thing is to admit the patient to the hospital. Roughly 30% of hospital stays in the United States are probably unnecessary given what this research demonstrates. And once someone is admitted, he or she is likely to be seen by a dozen or more specialists who will conduct myriad tests, whether these are absolutely essential or not (CBS News, 2009).

Dartmouth researchers also report that Medicare's total spending for the last 2 years of life varies significantly in the amount, intensity, and cost of care provided to chronically ill patients at the top academic medical centers. This, of course, raises the possibility of the government saving large amounts of money depending on where the patients are. Spending for the last 2 years of life ranges from $93,842 at the University of California Los Angeles (UCLA) Medical Center to $53,432 at the Mayo Clinic's teaching hospital in Rochester, Minnesota. In between these high and low averages were John Hopkins Hospital, Baltimore, at $85,729, Massachusetts General at $78,666, and Cleveland Clinic at $55,333 (Pear, 2008).

The data for the last 6 months are even more compelling, with average Medicare costs ranging from a high of $52,911 at UCLA and a low of $28,763 at the Mayo Clinic hospital. Note that more than 90 million Americans have chronic illnesses such as heart disease, diabetes, and cancer. Of these, 70% will die from the chronic disease, and the majority of Medicare spending on these chronic illnesses is for hospital care in the last 2 years (Pear, 2008).

This and other studies demonstrate that more care, and more intensive care, is not necessarily better for the patients. It is definitely possible that chronically ill, dying Americans receive too much care. And this is more care than the patients and their family actually want or really benefit from. What appears to account for the variation in Medicare spending at the end of life is the volume of services rendered, not the price of the services. Certainly it is time to consider another option that would give the patient and family the closure and gentle release that are so often desired, in addition to being cost-effective for both the family and Medicare.

Even at its best, Medicare has cost restrictions. The Medicare program pays for 80% of the approved costs. The other 20% is the patient's responsibility, and here is where the burden begins. As people approach age 65 they receive instruction from Medicare regarding their upcoming benefits. Many people are elated and believe they have finally gotten "free" insurance. What a certain percentage of these people don't realize is that they must also buy a supplemental policy to pay for the remaining 20% of charges. These unfortunates generally find this out too late, after they begin receiving bills. Those who read and understand the fine print continue paying for and receiving their old insurance policy or buy some sort of new supplemental policy. Those who don't do this may end up among the ranks of the seriously underinsured or bankrupt. Exhibit 5.2 offers more food for thought.

Medicaid

Medicaid is state-funded medical insurance. To receive this form of coverage individuals meet with social service agencies who evaluate their ability to pay or purchase their own policy. If they are determined to be indigent, the state pays their medical bills. At best, their expenses are paid. At worst, the system is filled with inconsistencies. Oftentimes, Medicaid recipients seek more care than is necessary or have more duplication of services than other pay groups of patients.

Private Insurance

Fortunately, all people can enroll in Medicare on their 65th birthday. However, thousands of terminal patients never reach this anniversary. Most private policies have significant copays (20% to 50%). The situation is that once a person is hospitalized, no one on the medical staff knows or even cares about what insurance policy the patient has, if any, to pay for the cost of care. Tests and treatments are ordered with "cure" in mind. It is the unusual situation where a doctor even considers palliative or hospice care before exhausting the cure approach. By the time the medical team has "given up" saving the patient and relegated him or her to hospice, palliative, or futile care, the expense has often soared to the stratosphere. Many hundreds of these patients and their families face bankruptcy. What a most unpleasant aftereffect of hospitalization in the terminal phase of life.

No Insurance

The odd thing about people with no insurance is that they often end up financially better off than those with private insurance. Once they arrive at the hospital and the admission clerk discovers they have no insurance, social service gets to work and, more often than not, arranges to get these patients covered by Medicaid, thus alleviating them of any pay liability. Consider the difference between the Medicaid patient's and the private insurance patient's end cost. For the patient with no insurance who receives Medicaid, the cost is zero. A self-insured person with a million-dollar bill pays between $200,000 and $500,000 depending on the copay. Does this seem fair?

HOSPICE AND PALLIATIVE CARE CONSIDERATIONS

The U.S. Medicare hospice benefit has expanded considerably into the nursing home setting in recent years. Although hospice utilization is

EXHIBIT 5.2   Consider This

Connie L., age 69, a widow with no children, has only Medicare as her insurance. She is in an automobile accident and sustains multiple traumas. She makes it to the hospital. After multiple surgeries and days in the intensive care unit (ICU), Connie asks to be let go. She wants to die, but due to heroic medical interventions, she survives and is transferred to a nursing home. Connie receives a hospital and doctor bill of $1 million for her ICU inpatient experience. Let's say that Medicare approves it all and pays 80%, or $800,000. Connie is now totally responsible for her $200,000 copay. What would you do? What can Connie do? Who pays? If Connie can't pay, what happens then? Is this what we want for our society? Should people be allowed to make their own end-of-life choices?

Unfortunately, this is how many Americans die. Roughly 18% to 20% of the terminal elderly spend their last days in an ICU. It's extremely expensive and very uncomfortable. Most patients have to be sedated so that they don't reflexively pull out a tube. To prevent this sometimes their hands are restrained. This is not the way most people would want to spend their last days of life. And yet this has become almost the medical last rites for people as they die.

Modern medicine has become so adept at keeping the terminally ill alive by treating the complications of underlying disease that the inevitable process of dying has become much harder and is often prolonged unnecessarily. Many families cannot imagine that there could be anything worse than having their loved one die. But, in fact, there is something worse. It's having someone you love die badly. How do so many people end up in the hospital? It's the path of least resistance.

Adapted from CBS News (2009).

relatively modest, its increased availability holds great promise. To date, there has been little research comparing hospice costs, service intensity, and quality of care across settings, reflecting the fact that few comparative data have been available to researchers. The Centers for Medicare and Medicaid Services have taken steps toward collecting these data, and further research is needed to shed light on what refinements, if any, are necessary for the Medicare hospice program (Taylor, 2009).

Words of Wisdom

> "Health care delivery in the United States and abroad has undergone tremendous growth over the last several decades. Accompanying this growth in the diagnostic and therapeutic armamentarium, the costs of health care have escalated out of proportion to the rest of the economy. This exuberant growth has engendered careful scrutiny of the practice of medicine with regard to both its effectiveness and its efficiency. This movement demands that physicians understand not only the effectiveness but also the cost of their interventions. Cost-effectiveness and cost–utility analyses have become critical evaluative tools in medicine. Explicit articulation of comparative cost-effectiveness is helpful in making choices about allocating limited resources in the setting of increasing competition for these resources."

From Zilberberg (2010).

One study examined the effect of the Medicare hospice benefit on Medicare and Medicaid expenditures by dual-eligible Medicare–Medicaid nursing home (NH) residents. Hospice enrollment results in substantial savings for the government (22% percent) among all short-stay (90 days or less), dying NH residents. For long-stay (greater than 90 days), dying NH residents, hospice provides some savings (8%) among cancer residents, while it is cost-neutral for dementia residents and adds some cost (10%) for residents with a diagnosis other than cancer or dementia. Hospice enrollment results in lower combined Medicare/Medicaid expenditures in the last month of life, particularly among short-stay NH residents. This effect, however, varies by diagnosis and NH length of stay. In addition, for short-stay NH residents, current payment policy creates a Medicare incentive and Medicaid disincentive for promoting residents' referral to hospice (Gozalo, Miller, Intrator, Barber, & Mor, 2008).

There is also the question of choosing hospice and its cost when compared with Medicare and more traditional end-of-life care. One study reviewed both types of costs in the United States with interesting results. Hospice is a rare example of an institution that offers quality end-of-life care while at the same time decreasing the costs of third-party insurers with multiprofessional interventions. Although out-of-pocket expenses appear to remain fairly consistent from hospice to hospice, the family incurs a number of informal expenses. The more personal, intimate time with the dying person would appear to compensate for the additional costs; however, these are difficult to measure. The Medicare program is established to offer essential and realistic care to beneficiaries. Hospice effortlessly passes this requirement (Payne, Coyne, & Smith, 2002). Since hospice is not accessible to nor used to a great extent by the large majority of the population, *Golden Rooms* seem a very reasonable option in hospitals and nursing homes for end-of-life care.

Questions have also been raised about costs and the efficacy of integrating palliative with curative modes of care earlier in the course of disease for people with life-threatening illnesses. On clinical grounds, initiating palliative care before people are actively dying is the mode, not the exception. The question and challenge are, What is a better, more cost-effective mode of care? All health care institutions, large or small, have asked this question. Some documentation is available for initiatives in larger hospitals and medical centers. If a palliative care consultation service is established, then costs are easily documented. At Memorial Sloan-Kettering Cancer Center in New York City, three simple potential cost-saving palliative care program models were piloted in their hospice program. They found that these simple models did not capture the cost savings that they had envisioned (Passik et al., 2004). Certainly within hospice adding palliative care appeared to improve and make care more efficient; however, the more complex patients also meant a shorter length of stay and increased drug costs, in addition to increased outpatient, emergency, and physician visits. The losses related to the palliative care program were being taken up by hospice.

Enter the *Golden Room*. Here the costs are minimal as comfort measures including pain medication are freely given and persons are allowed to make the transition in peace without the often frantic lab work, diagnoses, and treatments to sustain life. Comfort measures and in-room sleeping suites are available to the family, thereby reducing their financial burden too.

Only a few studies have assessed the economic outcomes of palliative therapy (Payne et al., 2002). Notice that this is palliative therapy, not palliative nursing care. Palliative care includes such things as

- Hospice care
- The process and structure of care
- Symptom management
- Palliative chemotherapy

- Ongoing lab tests
- Treatments and medications
- Surgery (Payne et al., 2002)

Most interesting is that hospice care saves at most 3% of total care costs when compared with traditional care (Payne et al., 2002). Advance directives done early in the disease course may save end-of-life care costs, but when done in the hospital they generally do not save money or influence care choices. Nurse coordination of palliative care maintained dying patients' clinical outcomes and saved 40% of costs. A structured ethics review of those likely to die in the intensive care unit also appears to match the type of care to the outcome and save costs. There are remarkably few randomized clinical trials of pain and symptom-control interventions in end-of-life care, so few conclusions can be drawn about current treatments (Exhibit 5.3).

Current data suggest that changes in palliative care costs can come only from dramatic changes in how we provide care. One model is coordinated, expert, high-volume care that can prevent end-of-life hospitalization, with early use of advance directives. Preliminary data from the program in this study support the hypothesis that costs may be reduced by 40% to 70% (Payne et al., 2002).

Worldwide agreement exists that aging societies will require more money for end-of-life care within already stretched health care budgets. This, coupled with the lower availability of family for informal care, means that a crisis of great proportion is looming. Currently there are 8,000 dedicated palliative care services worldwide (Gomes, Harding, Foley, & Higginson, 2009). This is a drop in the bucket compared to the need that is rapidly approaching. Because there has been no complete cost breakdown for palliative care, there are huge, looming questions that cannot be answered.

Even think tanks such as the international meeting in London in November 2007 are grappling with these issues. A group of 40 researchers, health economists, policymakers, and advocates exchanged their experiences, concerns, and recommendations in five main areas: shared definitions, strengths and weaknesses of different payment systems, international and country-specific research challenges, appropriate economic evaluation methods, and the varied perspectives on the costs of palliative care. Their views reflect the best research approaches to capture, analyze, and interpret data on both costs and outcomes for families and patients toward the end of life (Payne et al., 2002).

EXHIBIT 5.3   Point of View

There are no examples of chemotherapy that save money compared to the best supportive care. We must continue to ask whether the extended time really adds to the quality of life and whether it is worth the cost? If we don't ask this question, who will?

Our neighbors to the north, the Canadians, are also concerned about end-of-life costs as they expect their elderly population to double in 20 years (Chochinov & Kristjanson, 1998). They too have analyzed the literature regarding costs of this care and different models of care. The consistent themes and conclusions from their reviews were

- Depending on the model of care, costs of end-of-life care are considerable.
- Costs of care increase with distance from the home setting.
- Cost savings reported in palliative care settings may be a function of nearness to death.
- Family expenses for end-of-life care are substantial and are not factored into most cost analyses.
- A two-tiered system of palliative home care allows families with higher incomes to afford help in supporting home deaths.
- Some treatments given to dying patients are costly while yielding little benefit (Chochinov & Kristjanson, 1998).

Can we afford to wait another 20 or even 10 years when there are already early prototypes of the *Golden Room* in existence? Certainly in many ways we have missed the mark by not even bearing in mind that many, if not most, people would prefer to die surrounded by loved ones in a warm, loving environment without all the tubes, testing, and life-saving measures. It is time to not just reflect on but actively begin to listen to our hearts and think about how we want our loved ones to die, how we want to die, and what legacy we want to leave for our children and grandchildren. It is time for a place for death with dignity: the *Golden Room*. Consider the costs of waiting.

CONSIDERING LONG-TERM
HEALTH CARE POLICIES

A survey of 7,600 elderly in 1986 noted that elderly women have a less healthy last year of life as compared to elderly men. It demonstrated that 14% of all who died after age 65 were fully functional, while 10% were severely restricted. As age progressed, the statistics obviously got worse. Of those between the ages of 65 and 74, 20% were fully functional, while only 3% were severely restricted. At age 85, only 6% were fully functional, while 22% were severely restricted. Of particular note is that women were 40% less likely than men to be fully functional in the last year of life and 70% more likely to be severely restricted. Therefore, more women should consider long-term health care policies, and all should have durable powers of attorney for health care (Moody, n.d.).

SUMMARY

End-of-life care is in need of massive improvement, yet despite how much we know we still have scant information about the effectiveness or cost of various end-of-life therapies. It is likely that methods for conducting cost-effectiveness analyses for end-of-life care will need to evolve, or alternative strategies such as cost–benefit analysis or distributive justice will be needed to inform resource allocation decisions.

As the national debate about health care costs, access, and quality continues, we will increasingly turn to economic analyses to help make resource allocation decisions. Cost-effectiveness analysis will continue to be the most popular form of economic analysis because it combines the effectiveness of treatment with the costs of achieving the results (Pronovost & Angus, 2001). This includes discovering the costs and consequences associated with interventions aimed at reducing mortality and morbidity of critically ill patients at the end of life (Thomas, 2009).

REFERENCES

Barnato, A. E., Chang, C. C., Farrell, M. H., Lave, J. R., Roberts, M. S., & Angus, D. C. (2010). Is survival better at hospitals with higher "end-of-life" treatment intensity? *Medical Care, 48*(2), 125–132.

Buntin, M. B., & Huskamp, H. (2002). What is known about the economics of end-of-life care for Medicare beneficiaries? *Gerontologist, 42*(3), 40–48.

CBS News. (2009). *The cost of dying.* Retrieved May 3, 2010, from http://www.wkrg.com/financial/article/the_cost_of_dying/541220/Nov-23-2009_12-07-pm/

Chochinov, H. M., & Kristjanson, L. (1998). Dying to pay: The cost of end-of-life care. *Journal of Palliative Care, 14*(4), 5–15.

Emanuel, E. J. (1996). Cost savings at the end of life. What do the data show? *Journal of the American Medical Association, 275*(24), 1907–1914.

Fassbender, K., Fainsinger, R. L., Carson, M., & Finegan, B. A. (2009). Cost trajectories at the end of life: The Canadian experience. *Journal of Pain Symptom Management, 38*(1), 75–80.

Gomes, B., Harding, R., Foley, K. M., & Higginson, I. J. (2009). Optimal approaches to the health economics of palliative care: Report of an international think tank. *Journal of Pain Symptom Management, 38*(1), 4–10.

Gozalo, P. L., Miller, S. C., Intrator, O., Barber, J. P., & Mor, V. (2008). Hospice effect on government expenditures among nursing home residents. *Health Services Research, 43*(1, Pt. 1), 134–153.

McCrone, P. (2009). Capturing the costs of end-of-life care: Comparisons of multiple sclerosis, Parkinson's disease, and dementia. *Journal of Pain Symptom Management, 38*(1), 62–67.

Moody, E. F. (n.d.). *High cost of dying.* Retrieved May 18, 2010, from http://www.efmoody.com/longterm/dying.html

Passik, S. D., Ruggles, C., Brown, G., Snapp, J., Swinford, S., Gutgsell, T., et al. (2004). Is there a model for demonstrating a beneficial financial impact of initiating a palliative care program by an existing hospice program? *Palliative Support Care, 2*(4), 419–423.

Payne, S. K., Coyne, P., & Smith, T. J. (2002). The health economics of palliative care. *Oncology (Williston Park, NY), 16*(6), 801–808.

Pear, R. (2008). Researchers find huge variations in end of life treatment. *New York Times.* Retrieved May 14, 2010, from http://www.nytimes.com/2008/04/07/health/policy/07care.html?scp=4&sq=2008/04/07 &st=cse

Pronovost, P., & Angus, D. C. (2001). Economics of end-of-life care in the intensive care unit. *Critical Care Medicine, 29*(2, Suppl.), N46–N51.

Stevenson, D. G., & Bramson, J. S. (2009). Hospice care in the nursing home setting: A review of the literature. *Journal of Pain Symptom Management, 38*(3), 440–451.

Talmor, D., Shapiro, N., Greenberg, D., Stone, P. W., & Neumann, P. J. (2006). When is critical care medicine cost-effective? A systematic review of the cost-effectiveness literature. *Critical Care Medicine, 34*(11), 2738–2747.

Taylor, D. H. (2009). The effect of hospice on Medicare and informal care costs: The U.S. experience. *Journal of Pain Symptom Management, 38*(1), 110–114.

Thomas, E. (2009, September 21). The case for killing Granny. *Newsweek,* 37–38.

Zilberberg, M. D. (2010). Understanding cost-effectiveness in the ICU. *Seminars on Respiratory and Critical Care Medicine, 31*(1), 13–18.

6   *Legal and Ethical Issues*

When man forgot the real meaning of life then came law and order.
    —Chinese proverb

GRANDMA JAYNE'S STORY   Grandma Jayne had been fun loving, basically healthy, and attentive to her self-care all of her long life. During her early 90s she became incapacitated, so the family began to explore new options. Her granddaughter was the only relative to offer to bring Grandma to her home, which worked for awhile, but after a few months, the family decided Grandma's presence just wasn't a good fit. Grandma took out her dentures at the dinner table and set them in the salad bowl, she had toileting accidents on the couch, and her 8-year-old and 10-year-old great-granddaughters were beginning to bicker since one had given up her room and the girls had to sleep together to make space for Grandma. Finally it was decided to pack up Grandma and take her to a nursing home.

Grandma's stay went well at the nursing home for several years. Her family spent down all her saved money paying the nursing home bills while she aged into her 90s. Responsible granddaughter Linda had obtained durable power of attorney and a Do Not Resuscitate (DNR) order from Grandma Jayne's doctor during her routine care.

The month Grandma Jayne turned 97, her condition further deteriorated. Within a week, it was evident that her days were numbered. Then the problems began. When she stopped eating and became lethargic, the nursing home staff became insistent that they send her to the hospital. When Linda refused to have Jayne transferred, the staff then insisted that she have more care. Linda left work and came to the nursing home to see for herself. She arrived just in time to find the staff on the way to Jayne's room ready to insert a feeding tube. She stopped them outside the door to the two-bed room and refused to let them in. It is a well-established fact that once a feeding tube is inserted it is nearly impossible to get it removed. In Jayne's case her eyes were still open but there was no response to sound or physical stimulation.

Linda's blocking the door and forbidding the nurse to enter was a shock not only to the staff but to herself. She insisted that the nurse call the doctor and also that the nurse refer to the chart where it was posted that Jayne was a DNR patient. Eventually, the nurse acquiesced and the feeding tube was not inserted.

For the next 24 hours Linda and her family kept vigil at Jayne's bedside. They offered her sips of water, cleansed her mouth and brow, and allowed the staff to turn and clean her. Crammed into a small space between the window and the patient in the bed by the door, they made the best of their semiprivate room using a closed curtain around Jayne's bed. The next day, Grandma Jayne took her last breaths and made her transition into the next life.

Linda and her family went home exhausted. Grandma Jayne was gone and Linda was satisfied that she had made Jayne's passing as peaceful as possible.

REFLECTIONS ON ISSUES OF CONCERN

1. Should feeding tubes be mandatory for dying patients?
2. Should Jayne have been a candidate for a feeding tube?
3. What purpose do heroics play in the passing of terminally ill, elderly persons?
4. Was this the best setting for Jayne and her family during the dying process?
5. Was this setting helpful or disturbing to the family member who sat with her grandmother during this final phase?
6. Could something else have been done to make Jayne's transition more peaceful and loving?

LEGAL AND ETHICAL CONSIDERATIONS

Multiple challenges often arise with end-of-life decision making such as feeding tubes, nutrition, and life-sustaining machines yet, the major issue for many people is whether or not to forgo any life-sustaining medical treatment. When all else fails people or their families rely on the judicial system to solve the problem. In 1975, the first end-of-life case of national notoriety was the Karen Ann Quinlan case; the next, in 1998, was the Terri Schiavo case.

Karen Ann Quinlan Case

In the case of Karen Ann Quinlan, here was a young woman in what her doctors said was a state of unconsciousness from which she would never emerge. Although she was not dead, her parents believed, as did most people, that her life was over. From time immemorial, when this has occurred, we have allowed people in this type of permanent vegetative state to simply die. But Ms. Quinlan's doctors, for a variety of reasons given the era in which these events occurred, would not, in effect, permit this to happen. Her parents were denied the opportunity to allow her to normally pass away and then to mourn their loss in a culturally and religiously appropriate way. She was kept alive with modern medicine and all its contemporary trappings.

Her parents had two choices: accept the physicians' directives to keep her alive on life support, a direct affront to their values, their beliefs, and their dignity, or fight it. They fought it as long as they could through conventional means, but when those ultimately failed, they could continue to fight only by resorting to litigation. Litigation, however, has a number of limitations that ultimately make it a very unsatisfactory weapon in the armamentarium of solutions to end-of-life disputes.

In the litigation of end-of-life cases, like many other kinds of cases, the battle does not end the war. In all cases, the judicial decision, strictly speaking, applies only to that case. Everyone other than the parties to the case is entitled to ignore the decision. What happens in fact is far more complex than either uniform acquiescence or uniform defiance. Every litigated case in which an opinion is written by the court raises far more questions than it answers. And the bottom line is that nothing is solved for society as a whole.

Terri Schiavo Case

In the Terri Schiavo case, litigation went on for years beginning in the Florida courts and proceeding all the way up to federal court. Ms. Schiavo's ex-husband wanted to allow the persistent vegetative state woman to expire without the aid of artificial means, a feeding tube, and her parents did not.

Given the routine treatment of such right-to-die cases by state courts, Congress's extraordinary and last-minute intervention in the case attracted nationwide attention. At the conclusion of exhaustive litigation that resulted in the removal of life-sustaining treatment from an incapacitated patient pursuant to the directive of her surrogate husband,

Congress authorized federal jurisdiction over the Schiavo dispute. In response to this remarkable authorization, federal courts exercised customary deference to Florida's courts by refusing to issue a preliminary injunction to continue treatment and by declining to reexamine the settled state law issues. The federal courts' deference to the decisions of the state court precluded an examination of the constitutionality of Congress's allocation of federal jurisdiction and created another sensation in the right-to-die preference (Meisel, 2005). Many agree that Congress's anomalous action in the Schiavo litigation that negated her right to die should be viewed as a mistake not to be repeated in future end-of-life disputes (Rahdert, 2006).

As a result of these and a host of other cases, many end-of-life litigation cases emerged with the same arguments presented repeatedly in different courts. When we believe that the disputed solution cannot be solved in a rational, logical way and in our favor, many Americans jump to litigation. Einstein (n.d.) reminds us that "a problem cannot be solved at the same level of consciousness that created it."

LEADING ETHICAL ISSUES

There are a number of legal and ethical issues surrounding the right to die. Table 6.1 highlights the primary ones. Each of these ethical issues condenses to the questions of what does the dying person and the family desire and what does the medical community recommend and sometimes demand. Certainly when there are advance directives these decisions are usually simple—in theory (see chapter 2). The human emotional factor is always a huge consideration and often the determining factor.

The case of terminal sedation, as one example of the effect of the emotional factor, is now explored more fully.

Terminal Sedation: The Ongoing Debate

There has been much discussion regarding the acceptable use of sedation for palliation and/or end-of-life care. This hotly contended practice concerns deep, continuous sedation given to patients who are not imminently dying, without provision of hydration or nutrition, with the end result that death is hastened. This has been called *early terminal sedation*. Early terminal sedation is a practice composed of two legally and ethically accepted treatment options. Under certain conditions, patients have the right to reject hydration and nutrition, even if these are life-

TABLE 6.1   Legal and Ethical Issues at End of Life

Ethical issue	Definition
Resuscitation	Does the patient want cardiopulmonary resuscitation? Is it indicated? Should it be done on end-of-life patients?
Mechanical ventilation	What are the indications for being placed on a ventilator? Is this an acceptable procedure for end-of-life patients?
Nutrition and hydration	Should the patient be artificially fed? If this is determined feasible, for how long should it continue? When should nutrition and hydration be discontinued on a terminal patient? Should feeding tubes be inserted without permission? What are the long-term consequences? When can feeding tubes be withdrawn?
Antibiotics	Are antibiotics indicated at end of life? Pneumonia used to be termed the "old man's friend," as so many elderly ill succumbed to the disease. Often now, patients are put on antibiotic treatments even though they may be categorized as futile care patients.
Dialysis	When, if at all, is dialysis indicated in patients with terminal kidney disease? Does it matter if this treatment evolves from a temporary measure into a permanent event? When is it appropriate to end dialysis and offer palliative end-of-life care?
Terminal sedation	Use of deep, continuous sedation, often referred to as *double effect*. When is this indicated? Can one choose it for his or her own self? Who can administer?

sustaining. Patients are also entitled to sedation as palliation for intolerable, intractable suffering. Though early terminal sedation is thought to be rare at present, the changing nature of palliative medicine suggests its use will increase (Cellarius, 2009).

An examination of the literature reveals there are different definitions and explanations of terminal sedation. Some definitions appear compatible with the values of palliative care and nursing, whereas others could arguably be perceived as deserving of the term *euthanasia in disguise*. Some suggest that *palliative sedation* is a more helpful term and argue that, when defined and understood appropriately, it is a defensible and ethical practice. During these debates nurses should be clear about their purpose and honest about their intentions. They must respect the autonomy and dignity of the patients for whom they provide care. Generally, the doctrine or principle of *double effect* is the terminology used to support the practice of terminal sedation (Gallagher & Wainwright, 2007).

The debate continues as others see palliative sedation (sedation to unconsciousness) as an option of last resort for intractable end-of-life distress. This continues to be the subject of ongoing discussion and debate as well as policy formulation. A particularly controversial issue has been whether some dying patients experience a form of intractable suffering *not* marked by physical symptoms that can reasonably be characterized as existential in nature and therefore would not be an acceptable indication for palliative sedation. Such is the position recently taken by the American Medical Association. Some argue that such a stance reflects a fundamental misunderstanding of the nature of human suffering, particularly at the end of life, and may deprive some dying patients of an effective means of relieving their intractable terminal distress (Cassell & Rich, 2010).

As in the preceding argument, it is often claimed that the intentions of physicians are multiple, ambiguous, and uncertain, at least with respect to end-of-life care. This claim provides support for the conclusion that the principle of double effect is of little or no value as a guide to end-of-life pain management. Jansen argues that proponents of the claim fail to distinguish between two different senses of the word *intention*, and as a result are led to exaggerate the extent to which clinical intentions in end-of-life contexts are ambiguous and uncertain. Physicians, like others who make life-and-death decisions, have a duty to state clearly what their intentions are. Finally, the author argues that even if the principle of double effect should be rejected, clinical intentions remain ethically significant because they condition the meaning of extraordinary clinical interventions, such as that of palliative sedation (Jansen, 2010).

Some say that arguments regarding early terminal sedation have failed to recognize *early* terminal sedation as a distinct legal and ethical entity. It can be seen as both the simple sum of treatment refusal and sedation for palliation, analogous to terminal sedation. It can also be seen as an indivisible palliative treatment, more analogous to assisted suicide or euthanasia. But ultimately, it is wholly analogous neither to terminal

EXHIBIT 6.1   Point of View: Ethical Considerations

E thical considerations are crucial to any research study involving human participants, but particularly so when dealing
with participants who are 'as vulnerable as those in a palliative
care setting.

From Whiting and Vickers (2010).

sedation given when death is imminent, nor to assisted suicide or euthanasia. Cellarius (2009) contends that *early* terminal sedation should be
considered as a distinct entity. Such a reconception promises to provide
a way forward in the debate, practice, and policy regarding this conten-
tious area of palliative/end-of-life care.

What we do know is that advance care planning becomes an opportunity to extract the patient from the medical context and allow him or
her to speak about approaching death with close ones in his or her own
terms of reference. To this end, there is a need for facilitation of an intimate encounter where patients can speak about their concerns with their
loved ones (Shalev, 2010). One point of view is expressed in Exhibit 6.1.

ETHICAL POSITION STATEMENTS

The American Geriatrics Society has developed a number of ethical position statements to guide practitioners as they care for dying patients.
Additional positions are taken on the delivery and payment for care.
The salient three positions having to do with care of patient are detailed
in Table 6.2.

The American Holistic Nurses Association ethical position statement
is another example of a nursing organization's statement. See Table 6.3.
This position and other ethical reference points are derived from *Holistic
Nursing: Scope and Standards of Practice* (Mariano, 2007).

All major nursing associations have formal ethical position statements
or papers that essentially recognize the respect, dignity, and worth of the
person and the person's family. It is time to not just write about ethics: It
is time to put our words into action with each patient and family and in
this instance with the dying person and his or her family. Certainly our
actions speak louder than our words.

TABLE 6.2   American Geriatrics Society's Ethical Position
Statements to Guide Practitioners Caring for Dying Patients

Position	Rationale
1. The care of the dying patient, like all medical care, should be guided by the values and preferences of the individual patient. Independence and dignity are central issues for many dying patients, particularly in the elderly. Maintaining control and not being a burden can also be relevant concerns.	Optimal medical care of all patients, not just those who are dying, rests on frank and sensitive communication between patients and physicians. For dying patients, this ordinarily entails recognition and discussion of the facts surrounding prognosis and the likely course with a palliative plan of care. Conversations must attempt to elicit and respond to the patient's needs. Physicians sometimes face the challenge of being asked to respect patient's choices, which may maximize the quality of life and independence at the expense of optimal safety. This tension requires particular thoughtfulness and sensitivity to each patient's needs and values. When the patient loses decision-making capacity, care should be guided by previous conversations as well as by written advance directives, if available. Decisions made by surrogates should be guided by the patient's known and previously expressed wishes.
2. Palliative care of dying patients is an interdisciplinary undertaking that attends to the needs of both patient and family.	In caring for dying patients, caregivers themselves must develop a broad array of knowledge, skills, and attentiveness to comprehensive care. In addition, whether or not the patient is enrolled in a formal hospice program, physicians most often should function as members of a team. The team may include nurses, social workers, home health aides, physical therapists, personal caregivers, chaplains, volunteers, and the patient's family. Each team member contributes the special knowledge and skills of his or her discipline to help meet the needs of dying patients. Together, team members provide care for the patient and assist the family in coping with the patient's dying and death. Family members, as defined by the patient, usually play a critical role in both providing care for dying patients and in making decisions for dying patients who have lost decision-making capacity. Providing support for the patient's family, including a period after the patient dies, is an important aspect of the care of dying patients.

(Continued)

TABLE 6.2 (*Continued*)

Position	Rationale
3. Care for dying patients should focus on the relief of symptoms, not limited to pain, and should use both pharmacologic and nonpharmacologic means.	Pain, anxiety, depression, dyspnea, constipation, and other symptoms can all be significantly ameliorated, if not eliminated, in the vast majority of dying patients. Symptoms should be treated as vigorously as is appropriate to the patient's situation and preferences to maximize comfort, even if the unintended effect of these efforts is, on rare occasions, the hastening of death.

From *Position statement on the care of dying patients*, by American Geriatrics Society, 2007. Retrieved May 18, 2010, from http://www.americangeriatrics.org

TABLE 6.3 The American Holistic Nurses Association Ethical Position Statement

Position on holistic nursing ethics

Holistic nurses hold to a professional ethic of caring and healing that seeks to preserve wholeness and the dignity of self and others (Standards of Holistic Nursing, Core Value 1.3).

Code of ethics for holistic nurses

The fundamental responsibilities of a nurse are to promote health, facilitate healing, and alleviate suffering. Inherent in nursing is the respect for life, dignity, and the rights of all persons. Nursing care should be given within a context mindful of the holistic nature of humans, understanding the body–mind–spirit connection. Nursing care is unrestricted by considerations of nationality, race, creed, color, age, sex, sexual preference, politics, or social status. Given that nurses practice in culturally diverse settings, professional nurses must have an understanding of the cultural background of clients in order to provide culturally appropriate interventions.

Nurses provide services to a diverse array of clients that may include individuals, families, groups, or communities. Each client should be treated as an active participant in his or her health care and should be included in all nursing care planning decisions.

When providing services to others, each nurse has a responsibility toward the client, coworkers, nursing practice, the profession of nursing, society, and the environment.

From *Holistic Nursing: Scope and Standards of Practice*, by C. Mariano (Ed.), 2007, American Holistic Nurses Association, Silver Spring. Retrieved May 18, 2010, from http://www.ahna.org/Resources/Publications/PositionStatements/tabid/1926/Default.aspx#P2 7

Words of Wisdom

"Many patients with terminal illnesses choose palliative care to relieve symptoms, improve the quality of their lives, and strive for a peaceful death. Professionals who serve dying patients need to recognize the importance of advance directives as part of a patient's decision to forgo curative treatment for palliative care."

From Feeg and Elebiary (2005).

It is of interest to know that in June 2000, Taiwan enacted the Natural Death Act, a fact only recently being discussed in the United States. This was the first law of its kind in Asia and essentially allows competent patients with terminal illness to complete an informed consent for DNR orders. The Taiwanese have decided that natural death is a right and have established the practice. Exhibit 6.2 details a research study focused on terminal care for cancer patients after the enactment of the Natural Death Act in Taiwan. The study investigates one of the ethical dilemmas of this new law.

EXHIBIT 6.2   Research Perspective

A multicenter study surveyed 800 physicians and nursing staff of oncology wards and hospices through a set questionnaire. A total of 505 respondents (63.1%) who took care of patients with terminal cancer were analyzed. The most frequently encountered ethical dilemmas were truth-telling and place of care, both of which were related to communication issues. Dilemmas related to clinical management were artificial nutrition and hydration and use of antimicrobial agents. Analyses revealed that a positive attitude about the Natural Death Act was negatively related to the extent of ethical dilemmas. Based on their data, researchers concluded that the enactment of the Natural Death Act in Taiwan would contribute to improving the quality of end-of-life care. They further believe that this kind of law should be adopted in other countries. They advocate educating and encouraging cancer care professionals to build positive beliefs toward the act.

From Chiu, Hu, Huang, Yao, and Chen (2009).

Also of interest is another Taiwanese study that concludes, "A provision of appropriate training for medical professionals appears to be a useful educational strategy, and this result shows that the Natural Death Act should be included in nursing school educational programs. In the future, more effort should be made to fulfill patients' expectations and to follow medical ethics guidelines" (Tsai et al., 2005, p. 232).

SUMMARY

In the latter half of the 20th century, Western medicine moved death from the home to the hospital. As a result, the process of dying seems to have lost its spiritual dimension and become a matter of prolonging material life by means of medical technology. The novel quandaries that arose led in turn to medico-legal regulation (Shalev, 2010). Despite advances in care of the dying over the last 20 years, many recalcitrant system-level barriers prevent high-quality end-of-life care that is consistent with clinical and ethical standards and reasonably adheres to patient and family wishes for care and compassion.

A major barrier to high-quality end-of-life care is the confusion about end-of-life care despite the fact that most deaths today result from long-standing chronic disease (Tilden & Thompson, 2009).

The important issues, larger than the legal-ethical issues, are spiritual: goodness, compassion, peace, dignity, and release. As we move into the larger place in consciousness we begin to live from our heart and feel from our heart and move from our heart. The mandate becomes, "Do what is right." This "right" comes from deep inner heart wisdom, not the wisdom of anger or fear that results in attack. Resultant to living a heartfelt life, the *Golden Room* becomes a dignified place of quiet, gentle release surrounded by loved ones and supported by compassionate caregivers.

To this end the *Golden Room* would have been an ideal solution for either Karen Ann Quinlan or Terri Schiavo and their families. Here each woman and her family could have been surrounded and enfolded in love and gentle caring while allowing her death to be one of peace, gentle dignity, and release rather than national news that left family embittered and lives shattered.

It is time to remember an ethic that embraces death as a natural part of life and supports rather than penalizes those who seek a good death. A good death can occur without tubes and gadgets, pain and sorrow.

It is something we need to reawaken to and support as a final, loving, litigation-free ritual.

There are people who disagree with this perspective, but there are others who feel this inner calling and longing to be nurtured in death, to once again have this rite of passage return to its importance. There is a welcoming of death as a natural part of the life process. Grief accompanies death, yes, but death can be surrounded with an incredible realization of the continuity of life.

Often in our zeal to make ourselves more comfortable with the inevitable or to avoid an unavoidable happening such as death, we attempt to control the uncontrollable and reduce our personal fears by creating laws to artificially extend life. Unconsciously this soothes or at least defers having to deal with our own mortality. Every time a person dies, especially a loved one, we are reminded of our own mortality.

Concomitant with the rapidly increasing technology it is also time to embrace the natural cycle of life in this moment, rather than fear the future, including death. Now is the time to embrace a place for death with dignity: the *Golden Room*.

REFERENCES

American Geriatrics Society. (2007). *Position statement on the care of dying patients.* Retrieved May 18, 2010, from http://www.americangeriatrics.org

Cassell, E. J., & Rich, B. A. (2010). Intractable end-of-life suffering and the ethics of palliative sedation. *Pain Medicine, 11*(3), 435–438.

Cellarius, V. (2009). Early terminal sedation is a distinct entity. *Bioethics* [Epub ahead of print]. American Nurses Association. Retrieved from http://www.ncbi.nlm.nih.gov/pubmed

Chiu, T. Y., Hu, W. Y., Huang, H. L., Yao, C. A., & Chen, C. Y. (2009). Prevailing ethical dilemmas in terminal care for patients with cancer in Taiwan. *Journal of Clinical Oncology, 27*(24), 3964–3968.

Einstein, A. (n.d.). *Brainy quote.* Retrieved May 10, 2010, from http://www.brainyquote.com/quotes/quotes/a/alberteins130982.html

Feeg, V. D., & Elebiary, H. (2005). Exploratory study on end-of-life issues: Barriers to palliative care and advance directives. *American Journal of Hospice and Palliative Care, 22*(2), 119–124.

Gallagher, A., & Wainwright, P. (2007). Terminal sedation: Promoting ethical nursing practice. *Nursing Standard* (Royal College of Nursing, Great Britain), *21*(34), 42–46.

Jansen, L. A. (2010). Disambiguating clinical intentions: The ethics of palliative sedation. *Journal of Medicine and Philosophy, 35*(1), 19–31.

Mariano, C. (Ed.). (2007). *Holistic nursing: Scope and standards of practice.* American Holistic Nurses Association, Silver Spring. Retrieved May 18, 2010, from http://www.ahna.org/Resources/Publications/PositionStatements/tabid/1926/Default.aspx#P2

Meisel, A. (2005). The role of litigation in end of life care: A reappraisal. *The Hastings Center Report.* Spec No: S47–S51.

Rahdert, M. (2006) *The Schiavo litigation: A case study for federalism. Temple Political and Civil Rights Law Review, 15,* 423. Temple University Legal Studies Research Paper No. 2007-13. Retrieved May 18, 2010, from http://papers.ssrn.com/sol3/papers.cfm?abstract_id = 984293

Shalev, C. (2010). Reclaiming the patient's voice and spirit in dying: An insight from Israel. *Bioethics, 24*(3), 134–144.

Tilden, V. P., & Thompson, S. (2009). Policy issues in end-of-life care. *Journal of Professional Nursing, 25*(6), 363–368.

Tsai, L. Y., Lee, M. Y., Lai, Y. L., Li, I. F., Liu, C. P., Change, T. Y., et al. (2005). Practical effects of educating nurses on the Natural Death Act. *Support Care Cancer, 13*(4), 232–238.

Whiting, L. S., & Vickers, P. S. (2010). Conducting qualitative research with palliative care patients: Applying Hammick's research ethics wheel. *International Journal of Palliative Nursing, 2,* 58, 60–62, 64–66, 68.

Part II

Theory and Practice

7 *Theoretical Frameworks*

Conscious caring allows us to restore the heart of nursing and health care through theory-guided philosophical practices of heart-centered love and caring as the foundation for healing.

—Jean Watson, 2009

FRANK'S STORY   Frank, 76, had had a good life. He served in the Merchant Marines in World War II and worked his way up to major, then became captain of a large tanker. He spent most of his life at sea. Although he had never smoked, he now had a progressive lung cancer diagnosed 1½ years ago from the asbestos so prevalent in the ships in the 1940s. With premier health insurance and a living will he considered himself ready to have a dignified death. Frank and Hannah, his girlfriend of many years, moved closer to his only living family, his nephew, Allen, and his nephew's wife, Louise, in the Northeast. He enjoyed being with family after all those years of nomadic sea life.

Within 6 months of his diagnosis Frank began to go downhill rapidly, becoming too much for Hannah to care for at home. His physician admitted him to the regional hospital for a full workup with multiple tests and retests, consultations with state-of-the-art techniques, and the latest research. His diagnosis was metastatic cancer with beginning-stage in situ in multiple organs. After a month he was released to a nursing home, exhausted and unable to catch his breath without oxygen. His pain level had increased, requiring a morphine pump. The nursing home gave Frank the increasing care that he now needed. Once Frank entered the nursing home he never got out of bed again. Daily Hannah took care of him, doing whatever she was allowed to do. Despite the alternating mattresses and turning, Frank soon developed decubiti on his buttocks in addition to pressure sores on his elbows. His body was breaking down as his cancer spread to all areas of his body. Frank had a strong constitution. Even with multiple IVs, the morphine pump, and a failing body, day after day he kept on going.

After 16 months of steady decline, the nursing home personnel could no longer clean the decubitus ulcers on his buttocks because of their depth, and it was necessary to send him to the hospital via ambulance. Skin and bones and barely breathing, he was whisked to the regional hospital to get the best care. The debridement was painful, the ulcers now the size of baseballs on both hips. Although the living will was on his chart, the physicians continued to give him the best care he needed to stay alive. His nephew, Allen, was notified of this hospitalization and at 2:00 a.m. arrived with his wife, Louise, quite upset as to Frank's condition and what was being proposed. Since Frank was conscious, he was still being asked to determine his treatment and weakly just agreed to everything. After the debridement, Frank was returned to the nursing home by ambulance. The nephew, now aware of the severity of Frank's condition, flew into action and became Frank's health care power of attorney. This was an uphill struggle after all the time without one. One month later the nursing home called to have Frank sent to the hospital for debridement; the buttocks decubiti were now even larger. The nephew refused with one statement, "He is dying, let him die." Four days later, with Hannah, Bob, and Anne by his side, Frank died, having received the best treatment, the best technical care.

REFLECTIONS ON ISSUES OF CONCERN

1. What theory of nursing best describes the care that Frank was receiving and why?
2. How would Florence Nightingale interpret his care and progress?
3. How would the theory of either integral nursing or the theory of caring have changed the management of Frank's care?
4. How might the nurse assess how Frank and Hannah were coping on the painful, long-term process based on grief theory?
5. Often the focus of grieving is on the family and the dying person is not considered. What techniques would you use with Frank to assist him to resolve his mortality?

Nursing care at the end of life is concerned with assisting those dying through comfort measures on all levels—body, mind, and spirit—to allow them to gain a sense of peace and pass into the next realm with as much grace and dignity as possible. Nursing as a profession has focused holistically on the dying person's experience. Nurses seek to promote a sense of well-being through environmental influences and social and spiritual support. Nursing theories assist in both clarifying nursing practice and guiding nursing interventions in meeting patients' needs (Frisch, 2009).

PRIMARY THEORIES

It is always useful to guide practice on the basis of a theoretical framework. Many theories work well with end-of-life care. A number of primary and supporting theories and theoretical frameworks are detailed in the following.

Theory of Transpersonal Caring

A number of theories support the concept of death with dignity and gently guide us to the clarity of seeing the growing need for expansion of loving and caring dying facilities. Perhaps the most overriding is Watson's caritas (cosmic loving consciousness) theory, also known as the theory of transpersonal caring. Jean Watson (2009) views *caring science* as the moral, theoretical, and philosophical foundation for nursing, leading to transformative personal and professional practices. Nursing's humanist characteristics united with a scientific knowledge base are conceptualized within transpersonal caring theory, first presented by Watson in 1979. Nursing and the main concepts of person, health, and the environment are carefully intertwined within this framework. *Nursing* is reconciled by "professional, personal, scientific, esthetic, and ethical human care transactions" (Watson, 1988).

Caring science is defined as encompassing a humanitarian, human-science orientation to human caring processes, phenomena, and experiences. It includes arts and humanities as well as science. A caring science perspective is grounded in a relational ontology of being-in-relation and a world view of unity and the connectedness of all. Transpersonal caring acknowledges the unity of life and connections that move in concentric circles of caring—from the individual, to others, to the community, to the world, to Planet Earth, to the universe (http://www.watsoncaring science.org/caring_science/definitions.html).

This theory certainly fits with transforming how we encounter and assist the patient at the end of life. When nurses take responsibility for advancing nursing, practitioners, patients, and systems alike can

**EXHIBIT 7.1   Watson's Human Caring Theory:
Ten Caritas Processes**

1. Embrace altruistic values and practice lovingkindness with self and others.
2. Instill faith and hope, and honor others.
3. Be sensitive to self and others by nurturing individual beliefs and practices.
4. Develop helping-trusting-caring relationships.
5. Promote and accept positive and negative feelings as you authentically listen to another's story.
6. Use creative scientific problem-solving methods for caring decision making.
7. Share teaching and learning that address the individual needs and comprehension styles.
8. Create a healing environment for the physical and spiritual self that respects human dignity.
9. Assist with basic physical, emotional, and spiritual human needs.
10. Open to mystery and allow miracles to enter.

From Watson Caring Science Institute (n.d.)

witness a revolution in nursing. Conscious caring allows us to restore the heart of nursing and health care through theory-guided philosophical practices of heart-centered love and caring as the foundation for healing (Watson, 2009). A 10-point caritas process guides the nurse's actions. Exhibit 7.1 enumerates Watson's ten caritas processes. In one study Watson's 10 caritas factors formed the basis of an instrument to measure nursing students' perceptions of instructor caring (Wade & Kasper, 2006).

Watson's theory of caring and caritas proposes that caring and love potentiate healing. Rendering care as a "Caritas nurse" has implications for integrating caring and love into patient care, and measuring the impact of caring on patient and operational outcomes (Persky, Nelson, Watson, & Bent, 2008). A shift toward human caring values and an ethic of authentic healing relationships is required as systems now have to value human resources and life purposes, inner meanings, and processes for workers and patients alike, not just economics alone (Watson, 2006b). This shift requires a professional ethos with renewed attention to practice that is ethics/values-based and guided by theory as well as evidence and economics (Watson, 2006c).

All of these outcomes relate to those rendering care to end-of-life patients. Within Watson's perspective she questions: How do we walk through life? How do we get our footing to bring the artistry of caring into our lives and work and world? What steps do we take that speak to who we are and our raison d'être? This perspective is grounded in Newman's health as evolving consciousness, Rogers's science of unitary being, Quinn's view of sacred space, and Watson's own caritas (cosmic loving consciousness) perspective as the highest form of consciousness and the infinite source of healing and wholeness (Watson, 2006d).

Within caring theory, the primary nursing consideration is the creation of a caring, intimate relationship with the person. For caring to occur the nurse must both observe and accurately interpret the person's subjective experience and also interact with the person such that a significant and meaningful relationship is maintained. When the nurse and the person come together in a truly transformational situation, both are changed. For Watson these are "caring moments" and implicitly bring the sum of the parts (nurse and person) of the encounter into a new, higher level of understanding and relationship. Realizing the individual's self-worth as a human being, Watson strongly feels that no person should be objectified and treated as an object. As such, unconditional acceptance and positive regard for each person are a cornerstone of her theory. This theory challenges nurses to offer personal relations based on quality and caring while advancing health through knowledge and appropriate intervention (Frisch, 2009).

Caring is a universal phenomenon that transcends both geographic and cultural boundaries (Rexroth & Davidbizar, 2003). Watson's theory of human caring has served as a framework in many different nursing situations. Caring theory effectively guides sustained, high-performance nursing leadership through grounding in the inward journey of self-reflection and growth (Pipe, 2008). With the refinement and deepening of the theory of transpersonal care, Watson now characterizes the theory as both a theory and a caring science. A science having caring as the essential quality is the "foundational disciplinary framework for all caring-healing professions, moving beyond nursing" (Watson, 2006a, p. 63). One of the assumptions of this new caring science is "an expanding unitary, energetic worldview with a relational human caring ethic and ontology as its starting point" (Watson, 2006a, p. 28). As transpersonal caring theory continues to evolve in clarity and depth, the true sacredness of caring becomes apparent. As nursing health professionals we walk on sacred ground, doing sacred work, with sacredness personified within the nurse and the person separately and collectively.

Theory of Integral Nursing

A new and exciting theory of integral nursing was recently born from the knowledge, background, and application of the principles of holistic nursing and other theories. This grand theory includes an integral process, worldview, and dialogues that is praxis—theory in action (B. Dossey, 2009).

> *An integral process is defined as a comprehensive way to organize multiple phenomenon of human experience and reality from four perspectives: (1) the individual interior (personal/intentional); (2) individual exterior (physiology/behavioral); (3) collective interior (shared/cultural); and (4) collective exterior (systems/structures).* (B. Dossey, 2009, p. 17)

Integral theory helps nurses shift to a deeper level of understanding about being human related to the preceding four dimensions of reality. An integral worldview examines values, beliefs, assumptions, meaning, purpose, and judgments related to how one perceives reality and relationships from these four perspectives. An integral understanding allows us to more fully understand the complexity of human nature and healing, thus lending itself well as we work with end-of-life patients.

Nightingale's Theory

Many beginning nurses shy away from theories because they seem too abstract and not immediately useful to the hands-on practice of nursing. Florence Nightingale's "theory" of nursing gleaned from her 19th-century writings is classic. "Every day sanitary knowledge, or the knowledge of nursing, or in other words, of how to put the constitution in such a state as that it will have no disease, or that it can recover from disease, takes a higher place" (Nightingale, 1946, Preface). Nightingale ascertained the first principles of nursing—careful observation and understanding of patient needs, which we know today as assessment and diagnosis.

Nightingale is in incredible example of not only comfort nursing but also the putting together of observations, testing them and then making a broader statement of what needs to be done to assist both nursing care and the healing process. This is the essence of research and theory building—to guide the nurse in more effective nursing practice.

Different theories are relevant at different times depending on the situation and those involved. Not being mutually exclusive, theories with common terms and concepts can and often are used together. So one could say that we are all nursing theorists, like Nightingale, as we observe and determine what needs to be done and how to do it. We are all always collecting information with all our senses. In essence, as in formal research, we as nurses consider the past and what has happened, look at the purpose, measure the incident, and then consider the action steps that we need to take for a preferred outcome. This sounds like the nursing process!

How appropriate is Nightingale's theoretical approach of observation and determining what needs to be done in caring for those dying and their families? Although many things can be predetermined there is still the unknown of what takes place in the present moment. It is here that we meet the dying person and the family and here that we must move from a place of deep knowing and from an open heart to respond to their immediate needs for comfort and care.

Nightingale taught what we now recognize as her theory in terms of ways of doing things or patterns of behaviors that nurses need to address in their care. This is the way many theories are taught. Another example of this, as suggested earlier, is the nursing process, which we know as a logical and specific format to clearly and easily determine care for all patients. In essence, nurses learn to assess, plan, treat, and then evaluate. This has evolved into a pattern of behavior that all nurses have learned and, we hope, apply to each patient.

Just as Nightingale considered the larger perspective or foundation of improving health care so present-day nursing theorists reflect on the theoretical basis of nursing practice as a discipline and as an art. Being specific to explain and direct nursing practice, these theories are often supported by larger, broad theories from other disciplines, such as general systems theory from science or phenomenological theory from philosophy. Since nursing theories are also considered broad they can have theories within them that reflect different aspects of patient care. Specifically, these theories can speak to various aspects of the end of life such as care, grief, and transcendence.

Holistic Nursing Theory

Holistically, the *person* is seen based on the knowledge that the whole is greater than and different from the sum of its individual components. As a subjective state determined by each person, *health* relates to feelings of harmony and unity, whereas illness is perceived as dissonance and separation from the whole. Based on elements provided in the *environment*, caring is perceived. These elements are social, cultural, and spiritual influences (Frisch, 2009). Holistic nursing is essentially caring for others within an ever-changing environment including body, mind, and spirit. The environment consists of one's own and the other's environment, both internal and external. The *internal environment* relates to

- Thought processes, mental status, and clarity
- The nature of one's own state of relaxation or tension
- The degree of "centeredness" within the caregiver and the patient
- Mental development and acuity of thought
- The nature of one's own spiritual development

The *external environment* relates to things in the physical setting, such as

- Air quality
- High noise level versus soothing, gentle sounds
- Comfortable seating or resting facilities
- Excess visual stimuli or calming color or scenes
- Intellectual milieu or setting where the interaction occurs
- Current cultural settings and acceptance of spiritual differences

"By definition and by history, nursing is a holistic practice. Nursing's work is concerned with . . . helping the client gain a subjective sense of peace and harmony" (Frisch, 2009, p. 113).

Two major challenges in nursing have emerged in the 21st century. The first is to integrate the concepts of technology and spirit into nursing practice; the second is to create and integrate models for health care that guide the healing of self and others. Holistic nursing is the most complete way to conceptualize and practice professional nursing (B. Dossey & Guzzetta, 2005, pp. 8–9). Many holistic nursing concepts are used in theory and practice. Interconnectedness and story are two examples offered here.

Interconnectedness

Interconnectedness reflects the fact that people and the universe are connected in a powerful way. Its essential meaning is that, regardless of the worldly barriers of politics, religion, or culture, people can share in a universal reciprocity of love and responsibility. Nursing maintains the values of compassion, responsibility, and holism. These ideals contribute to greater meaning of experiences with increased significance for practicing nurses (Love, 2008). Holistic nurses embrace the concept that the person and group are greater than the sum of the parts in a variety of ways. For example, using a group modality approach, a nurse can increase the number of people served. The group modality is a viable holistic treatment consideration for the elderly, given the steady increase in the elderly population, the presence of various psychiatric and/or medical conditions in this cohort, and cost concerns (Puskar, Brar, & Stark, 2008). Researchers Spence and Smythe (2008) argue that there is value in continuing to question the meaning of "being a nurse." Amid a complex and increasingly technological world, this repeated question calls the profession to remember the human encounter at the heart of all nursing (Spence & Smythe).

Use of Story

Holistic nursing as a process is contextually illuminated by creating a story within a story and believes that stories convey meaning and open us to the deep mystery of compassion. "Stories are methodological tools in the aesthetic domain of nursing, paratelic ways of knowing that carry us beyond logic to a higher order of understanding. Through stories we are connected to each other and to ourselves" (Repede, 2008, p. 226). The idea of story it that will open the reader or listener to his or her own unique understanding of the meaning of healing. Story can be used in sharing circles and other group processes to further people's understanding of letting go. Throughout this book the reader sees how we as authors use the holistic tool of stories at the beginning of each chapter to illuminate our concepts.

In addition to these major theories, there is validating research and a host of supportive theories that relate to compassionate end-of-life care. Exhibit 7.2 outlines one study.

SUPPORTIVE THEORIES

Grief Theory

Grief theory considers not only the grief process but also ways to assist the dying and their families to resolve their grief and move on in life. Although everyone experiences grief at some or numerous points in their lives, it is a powerful personal experience that, while having

EXHIBIT 7.2   Research Perspective

A recent study used a grounded theory approach to formulate a conceptual framework of the nursing role in end-of-life decision making in a critical care setting. Interviews were conducted with 14 nurses from intensive care and cardiorespiratory care units. The core concept, Supporting the Journey, became evident in four major themes: Being There, A Voice to Speak Up, Enable Coming to Terms, and Helping to Let Go. Nurses described being present with patients and families to help validate their feelings and give emotional support. Nursing work, while bridging the journey between life and death, imparted strength and resilience and helped overcome barriers to ensure that patients received holistic care. The conceptual framework challenges nurses to be present with patients and families at the end of life, clarify and interpret information, and help families come to terms with end-of-life decisions and release their loved ones.

From Bach, Ploeg, and Black (2009).

similar processes, is rather unique in its expression. This places the nurse in a very sensitive and pivotal position to give exceptionally personalized care for both the dying person and the family.

Grief Defined

The term *grief* is actually a general term that often incorporates other words or feelings, such as depression, bereavement, loss, and mourning. Each of these grief-related words has a subtle difference in meaning as explained in Table 7.1. Grief is often spoken of as an inner feeling of sadness caused by loss of a loved one, a pet, a significant other, or something special in one's life. Grief is not time bound. As the result of this loss, there is both mourning and bereavement, which are nuances of the same thing. *Bereavement* is a more specific type of loss involving the death of a significant other such as parent, child, spouse, or partner, while *mourning* is tied to cultural traditions and rituals. In the Jewish tradition the mirrors are covered and mourning lasts for one year. In many cultures black is the traditional color of mourning. The period of mourning varies from one culture and tradition to another and can vary from a few months to a year.

TABLE 7.1   Terms Related to Grief

Term	Meaning
Bereavement	An emotional response to loss of a person or thing
Depression	A normal stage of grief when not prolonged A clinical diagnosis often following loss Extended sadness
Loss	Absence of a significant person or thing
Mourning	An expression of sorrow, often sadness after a loss

Loss is a general term for grief and can be the consequence of a change in life or in one's circumstance in life. Many types of loss are a normal part of this physical existence and are usually taken in stride and can be adapted to rather well. Such losses are listed in Exhibit 7.3. More specific losses happen during the dying process, which can begin gradually and occur over an extended period of time or can take place quite rapidly. Either way the losses during the dying process are apparent not only to the dying person but also to the caretaker and family. The losses that occur during the dying process are seen in Exhibit 7.4. Many factors affect the response to loss in the grieving process, such as the nature of what was lost, the personal history of loss, and the familial structure and function, as well as the cultural rituals and customs.

EXHIBIT 7.3   Types of Losses Considered Part of Life

- Aging
- Amputation
- Disability/paralysis
- Divorce
- Empty nest
- Moving
- Retirement
- Loss of sexual intimacy
- Unemployment

EXHIBIT 7.4   Losses during the Dying Process

- Loss of control
- Loss of function
- Loss of sexual intimacy
- Loss of relationship

Major Grief Theories

Grief theory is very broad and encompasses a rich tapestry of concepts and ideas that assist the nurse in determining appropriate nursing care. As a theory, grief has multiple diverse origins beginning in psychoanalytic theory (Freud, 1957) and medicine (Lindemann, 1944; Kübler-Ross, 1969), expanding into psychology (Caplan, 1974) and finally into pastoral care (Kushner, 1981). Along the way many researchers have added their understandings and expanded the concepts.

In retrospect the decade of the 1960s appears to be significant as seminal theories of the stages of grieving were published then. Bowlby (1961) noted the four stages of grieving as protest, despair, detachment, and resolution. Eight years later, Kübler-Ross (1969) hypothesized the five stages of grieving as denial, anger, bargaining, depression, and acceptance. Then in 1975 Kübler-Ross incorporated developmental theory as she perceived the final stage of growth to be death.

Qualities of Grief

The highly individualized, ever-changing process of grieving has five qualities that appear to encompass all experiences within it: individualized, dynamic, pervasive, chronic, and normative. Each quality has within itself numerous other qualities or variables to consider. The whole process of grieving is complex although the stages appear simple and straightforward.

Individualized.   Grief is quite possibly one of the most studied and least understood processes that the nurse can experience, both personally and professionally. So many factors influence how each person responds to loss that it is almost impossible to predict. One person can be quite constrained and inward focused, while another can be demonstrative and outward focused. See Exhibit 7.5.

EXHIBIT 7.5   Variables Affecting Grief

- Cultural beliefs and rituals
- Nature of relationship with the deceased
- Previous losses
- Spiritual and religious background
- Support system available

Dynamic.   The nature of grief can be ever-changing and in a constant state of flux. Often there appears to be an ebb and flow of sensations, feelings, and thoughts that appear to be erratic and random rather than to form specific progressive stages. Grief is so dynamic that there is really no time limit to the process. Grief is simply the time each person takes to move into acceptance of the loss of a loved one. This can be weeks to months to years to a lifetime, and each is appropriate for that person. The first year especially appears to rekindle memories and loss at special times such as birthdays, the anniversary of the loss, the wedding day, or even Memorial Day and Veterans Day.

Pervasive.   Grief can often seem enveloping, persistent, omnipresent, invasive, and insidious, appearing in all areas of one's life. Grief can become so intense that physical symptoms may occur such as shortness of breath, cold sweats, palpitations, hyperventilation, and difficulty swallowing. Mentally, decision making becomes difficult, if not impossible. The bereaved often looks to family or friends to make decisions or simply does not make a decision. Even simple tasks such as fixing meals or sleeping become difficult. Acute grieving is not time bound and can occur or reoccur almost like a delayed reaction. When it arises, this feeling of "I can't go on" knows no boundaries in its level of acuity or level of frequency. It is simply there and appears to affect everything.

Chronic.   Grief may be experienced as chronic, with unexpected outbursts over very small things both during the dying process and even years later. A sudden outburst may occur at the thought of losing a loved one, and uncontrollable crying often feels unremitting and unending. Coming across one of Mother's lace hankies in a cedar chest, or finding Father's hammer among things to be given away can seem like unrelenting, constant reminders of the loss of a loved one. Even years later, an unexpected sudden occurrence of tears upon hearing a certain song or smelling the ocean can occur. At this point the tears and grief are usually short lived. What appeared to be chronic because it filled every minute of one's life in every area of life gradually lifts into cherished memories that can be felt and released into a greater sense of health and well-being. There is a gradual release and transformation into a new level of being and understanding.

Normative.   Although grief is accepted as a normal process that everyone goes through to a greater or lesser degree, cultures and societies have established expectations of what normal actually is—of what is acceptable. So what is considered normal within one culture would be considered pathological or atypical in another culture. Group norms are a type of culture that can also determine the acceptance or non-acceptance of how a person grieves. Often, however, the way a person grieves can be considered inappropriate. Consider the health care personnel in a hospital and their expectations of what is normal immediately after death. There also is an expectation that the family or significant others will make decisions about funeral homes, cremation, who to call, and possibly organ donations. There is an expectation that the family needs some time with the deceased, but not too long because the bed is needed for another patient. There is paperwork to complete and forms to sign and possibly an autopsy if indicated. The body needs to be prepared and removed from the floor as quietly and unobtrusively as possible. The family is expected to think clearly and have any information needed to complete this process. If there is too much crying and loud mourning the staff can feel uncomfortable and move to quickly quiet, calm, or even sedate the mourner to keep an air of decorum in the hospital setting. The opposite is also true. If the family is unresponsive and numb and shows no emotion, then the staff may perceive them as cold and uncaring. What is normal within the family can be seen as abnormal within the society at large.

Consequences of Grieving

Although grief has many facets and variables, everyone experiencing grief does attain two long-term results. All persons arrive at a new level of reality and new identity or sense of self. This applies to both the bereaved person and the dying person. For the bereaved person and family there is a new truth that their roles no longer include the deceased. Their day-to-day reality is forever changed. They can no longer call or see the deceased. They might have to take on new tasks that previously were taken care of by the deceased, such as balancing the checkbook, washing dishes, shoveling snow, or calling the repair person. There is no longer someone to talk things over with or to get an opinion from. New tasks are literally forced on the survivors, causing them to change, develop new roles, and expand their identity. As these daily truths become apparent, gradually a new sense of identity begins to emerge.

There are always choices, even for the bereaved. Moving into a new truth and new roles can be a gentle process of discovery in the moment, moving step by step, or a process of difficulty and refusal to accept what is. The latter keeps the bereaved stuck in continued grieving. Sadly, in America, if a person appears to be grieving too long, he or she is termed dysfunctional, which connotes a mental illness. Dysfunctional grieving is seen as the incapability to function properly in society.

In contrast to the bereaved person, the dying person has a finite amount of time and decreasing energy to arrive at a new reality and a new identity. The three clinical phases between the time the dying person recognizes the end of life and the moment of death were first described by Hess (1990) as acute crisis, chronic living dying, and terminal. Similar to the qualities of grief for the bereaved, these phases are also dynamic, pervasive, and individual and give nurses a form to support the dying person as he or she completes the tasks of dying. The nurse is responsible in all phases to generate a physical, mental, and emotional environment that supports the dying person both in controlling as much of the living dying process as desired and in cocreating relationships with family and friends (Hess, 1990).

In phase one, the acute phase, there is instability as the person, family, and friends become aware of the terminal prognosis. The nurse can assist them to refocus away from the terminal diagnosis into the present moment and deal with the small occurring losses as they arise. The nurse can be instrumental in supporting the denial–hope cycle and move those involved into a meaningful relationship in each moment so that they really live and enjoy life each moment. Crisis intervention is sometimes needed during this phase.

The chronic living-dying stage, phase two, can often continue for two to three years or longer. During this time the dying person physically integrates the needed therapies and treatments (e.g., stress tests, laboratory work, radiation, chemotherapy) into his or her present life.

The priority soon becomes evident upon completion of the "bucket list" of things that are important to do in this lifetime while preserving time and energy. Oftentimes alternative therapies are implemented, such as massage, imagery, meditation, and healing touch; these need to be encouraged by the health care professionals as they support the dying person holistically. A watchful eye needs to be kept on the amount of treatments and therapies engaged in so that they are supportive and do not become an exhausting list of things to do. Mentally, during phase two there are also tasks to be completed to bring the dying person to peace with his or her life and relationships with others. A life review is often completed and reflected upon. Family members often find that at this phase, simply being with the dying person, sharing, laughing, and many times simply sitting together quietly, is healing. Holding hands or touching is spontaneously and intuitively supportive of both the dying person and the family. Relationships and mending them are priorities at this time. Resolving old issues and saying good-bye gently and lovingly allow the dying person to feel that his or her life had dignity and meaning.

The terminal phase, phase three, is a time for the dying person to draw inward. Physical tasks have either been accomplished or discarded, and more physical assistance is needed. A space of gentle quiet is usually the mode, with talk being soft and easy and not requiring the dying person to interact. The hope for remission or a miracle turns to deep compassion and comfort in accepting what is—the natural completion of the life cycle.

Culture Theory

Ideas regarding culture as it pertains to nursing care and now to the end of life have been changing. First, in basic nursing education, a concern was often stated about being sensitive to differing cultures with respect to appropriate care. There was little emphasis or consideration on culture in the area of end-of-life care. This first began a quantum shift as Leininger (1978, 1991, 1998) pioneered the theory of *transcultural nursing*, which generally states that nursing care must be given with cultural awareness to be truly effective and meet the needs of the patient. This salient theory reflects the long-held holistic respect that nursing holds for the variations between people as well as the often widely divergent values that need to be integrated into nursing care. As a result cultural characterizations such as those that follow have evolved with respect to nursing care and culture:

- Cultural awareness: distinguishing the variation in beliefs, attributes, and values
- Cultural competence: the capacity to work successfully within a culture
- Cultural diversity: normal variations in attitudes, behaviors, and values depending on group membership; frequently associated with race or ethnicity
- Cultural sensitivity: an understanding that patients often have attitudes, behaviors, and values that differ from those of the nurse, along with a readiness to discover the differences (Olson, 2001)

Research in cultural competence and cultural sensitivity has been steadily increasing since Leininger first published her theory (see Table 7.2). In 2004, the Center for Nursing Research at the Johns Hopkins University School of Nursing examined research and theoretical literature to determine emerging themes surrounding factors influencing the integrity of the dying patient in an effort to develop a conceptual framework for continuing research. Going beyond previous frameworks for the end of life, their framework included the health professional and the health care organization's relationship to the integrity of the person. Outcomes added to the usual comfort and quality of life were the achievement of life goals and patient decision-making methods. Attention was focused on the cultural dimension of the dying person in a multicultural society. The definition of the end of life was also enlarged to take in both the frailty of heath in advanced age and terminal illnesses' acute phase (Nolan & Mock, 2004).

Over the last decade there has been increasing interest in transcultural spirituality together with nursing practice at the end of life and bereavement. Nursing literature has been in the vanguard of addressing

TABLE 7.2   Four Stages of Cultural Competence

Unconscious incompetence	No understanding of lack of comprehension of cultural issues
Conscious incompetence	Becoming aware of lack of comprehension of cultural issues
Conscious competence	Learning the pertinent cultural issues in giving care
Unconscious competence	Automatically responding with culturally congruent care with diverse cultures

culturally competent practice and the significance of patients' belief systems. In a review of the literature on both philosophical and spiritual issues surrounding death, dying, and bereavement, common themes and approaches offer a framework to guide nursing practice. A framework is even more germane to clinical practice; without guidance most nurses struggle in giving spiritual care because of its complexity and changeability. As a result nurses time and again resort to broad classifications (Holloway, 2006).

When culture is a core value, practitioners and researchers cannot assume that culture has been considered without stating how culture interacted with the phenomenon of concern. Core Value IV of the American Holistic Nurses Association includes valuing the client's cultural background.

As has become apparent, issues and theories surrounding culture and competence are still in their infancy and are very complex. Cultural competency is not a natural occurrence. Even within one's own familiar culture there are individual and family variances in beliefs and practices surrounding death and dying. The health care professional needs to become a culturally competent clinician. This does not require knowledge of or experience with every cultural belief and practice, but it does require, first, that one become sensitive to others' values and preferences, and, second, that one not assume that one person represents the values and preferences of the group. These, along with the underlying ability to be in the present moment and discover what is appropriate, instead of going on past experience or knowledge, open the nurse to listen and hear, to observe and see what is needed at this point in the dying process. This greatly enhances cultural competency as people are more willing to share their customs when they sense that the other is open and seeking to understand and not judge them. This genuine caring ensures that culturally competent care is effortlessly provided.

Self-Transcendence Theory

Self-transcendence is a term that has been used for years, usually referring to moving beyond one's self and into a wider place in consciousness and understanding. At the heart, it is a spiritual concept that we are continually expanding into a more aware nature as we acquire a deeper understanding of who we really are—our true self. Transcendence is a personal journey of self-discovery, and it involves personal effort and the willingness to learn and change. As such it can take a lifetime and is often associated with old age and the end of life, as that is when it frequently becomes more apparent. "The term came to nursing with a purpose . . . to enhance understanding about well-being in later adulthood. The theory is also applicable to any person whose life situation increases awareness of vulnerability and personal mortality" (Reed, 2008, p. 105).

The universal idea of transcendence being accomplished at the end of life is accepted since clients' well-being is repeatedly compromised with end-of-life issues (Reed, 1991). Self-transcendence appears to be a source for personal healing even when a cure is not possible. As one reaches beyond the self's boundaries, a sense of well-being often can become apparent. This presents itself through an intensified consciousness of integration and wholeness with all life and all dimensions of one's personal being (Coward & Reed, 1996).

Transcendence has been validated in many areas of nursing care and nursing situations. Depression in middle-aged adults has a significant inverse correlation with self-transcendence (Ellermann & Reed, 2001), as has also been demonstrated with AIDS memorial quilt makers (Kausch & Amer, 2007). Elderly nursing home residents who have a spirit of acceptance and serenity are able to transcend losses in later life and maintain more contentment and satisfaction in living (Bickerstaff, Grasser, & McCabe, 2003). Neill (2005) gives the stories of seven women living with multiple sclerosis or rheumatoid arthritis that demonstrate how, when health is viewed as expanding consciousness, self-transcendence into new ways of living such as being positive, gaining self-control, enjoying simple pleasures, and achieving self-differentiation can occur. Registered nurses on acute care staff demonstrated a significant positive correlation between transcendence and work engagement, with those with higher self-transcendence having more energy, dedication, and absorption in their work (Palmer, Quinn-Griffin, Reed, & Fitzpatrick, 2010). Self-transcendence seen as authenticity, reflective understanding, and consciously developed unity has even been demonstrated to assist in the incorporation of nursing practice, science, and theory (Perry, 2004).

Transcendence is often associated with spirituality in addition to old age and the end of life. An electronic literature search for research published from 1985 to 2003 examined spirituality as essential to a wisdom of meaning and life purpose that relates to the sacred or self-transcendence. The 13 studies reviewed showed that some spiritual aspects remain stable as one ages while other spiritual aspects, such as tasks, and needs of aging, change. Common spiritual themes running through the study consisted of changing relationships, integrity, concern for younger generations, humanistic concerns, and a growing relationship with a transcendent being, in addition to coming to terms with death, power, and their own transcendence. The findings were not related to age in years but rather to challenges inherent in aging (Dalby, 2006).

All dying persons do not necessarily accomplish self-transcendence. Still, all dying persons need to be sustained and nourished emotionally as they seek transcendence. It is here, in this search for transcendence, that all religions and spiritual practices come together on the common ground of going beyond the limitations of the self and becoming aware of something more, our higher source. Although called by many names this higher source lies beyond any metaphysical idea or concept. Transcendence is not limited to spiritual or religious persons. That is the beauty of it. Anyone working for greater excellence and a higher understanding is practicing a type of self-transcendence.

Transcendence replaces the old ideas of the self as contained and controlled by this physical mind and body with a vast self. The old boundaries and definitions fade away and former distinctions once thought so important no longer constrict. The realization comes that you are more, so much more than you can physically know or even imagine and the universe is indeed interconnected rather than separate. In this magnificence you are and have always been a piece of all that is. The universe is nonlocal, and instead you are everywhere and you are nowhere (L. Dossey, 2008, 2009). Only in the physical self in this physical life do you appear to inhabit only a small place in the grand design of things.

In the final analysis, striving for transcendence at the end of life, finding meaning and connectedness, helps make grieving less thorny and turns the inevitable into a reason for hope. Transcendence sometimes occurs at the very end of life just prior to death, called a *transcendent moment*, and appears as great joy and peace with clarity of countenance.

Certainly self-transcendence is also true for the caregivers—nurses, family, and friends—and can be found if they accept the feelings they are having and move into deeper awareness. Here, being in the present moment becomes powerful as everyone in the room looks inward, recognizes and feels the feelings that are present, stays connected with family and friends, and accepts the incredible space of timelessness as the death moment approaches. This is why family and loved ones automatically move into a *life review* as an unconscious way to see what was meaningful by simply remembering. Life review reserves a place in history for the dying person so that the hurt of loss in time can be replaced with a sense of cherishing.

Words of Wisdom

" $\mathbf{A}$ lthough Nightingale's legacy foresaw the rise of modern nursing in the 20th and 21st centuries, her enduring legacy is yet to be actualized; it reaches past this era and lures us into her prophetic vision that is already on us. Her vision of health and healing, of science and art, of the individual and the divine, of the natural, of nature and of the cosmos—now embedded in contemporary concepts and philosophies of transpersonal caring and healing practices—will carry us forward as a blue print through another century and beyond."

From Watson (2010, p. 108).

SUMMARY

Theories from the very simple to the very complex provide guidance and direction for effective nursing care for the dying and their families. Working from expected patterns of behaviors and putting theory into action assist the nurse to observe and assess needs based on where the dying and their families are and determine strategies to meet those needs. When the nursing process and theories come together in the present moment and move from an open heart, insightful, gentle, loving care is given and felt.

Self-transcendence is a powerful key for giving nursing care and also for assisting the dying and their families in the face of the inevitable. This feeling of connecting inwardly to one's deepest self and concomitantly outwardly in relationship with others helps everyone discover that life has meaning. This realization that all life has meaning further supports us to live fully in the present moment, finding joy and peace even in the shadow of death.

REFERENCES

Bach, V., Ploeg, J., & Black, M. (2009). Nursing roles in end-of-life decision making in critical care settings. *Western Journal of Nursing Research, 31*(4), 496–512.

Bickerstaff, K., Grasser, C., & McCabe, B. (2003). How elderly nursing home residents transcend losses of later life. *Holistic Nursing Practice, 17*(3), 159–165.

Bowlby, J. (1961). Process of mourning. *International Journal of Psychoanalysis, 42,* 317.

Caplan, G. (1974). Foreword. In I. Glick, R. Weiss, & C. Parkes (Eds.), *The first year of bereavement* (pp. vi–xi). New York: Wiley.

Coward, D., & Reed, P. (1996). Self-transcendence: A resource for healing at the end of life. *Issues in Mental Health Nursing, 17*(3), 275–288.

Dalby, P. (2006). Is there a process of spiritual change or development associated with ageing? A critical review of research. *Aging and Mental Health, 10*(1), 4–12.

Dossey, B. (2009). Integral and Holistic Nursing: Local to Global In B. Dossey & L. Keegan, *Holistic nursing: A handbook for practice* (5th ed., p. 17). Sudbury, MA: Jones and Bartlett.

Dossey, B., & Guzzetta, C. (2005). In B. Dossey, L. Keegan, & C. Guzzetta, *Holistic nursing: A handbook for practice* (4th ed., pp. 8–9). Sudbury, MA: Jones and Bartlett.

Dossey, L. (2008). Transplants, cellular memory and reincarnation. *Explore, 4*(5), 285–293.

Dossey, L. (2009). Mind–body medicine: Whose mind and whose body? *Explore, 5*(3), 125–134.

Ellermann, C., & Reed, P. (2001). Self-transcendence and depression in middle-age adults. *Western Journal of Nursing Research, 23*(7), 698–713.

Freud, S. (1957). Mourning and melancholia. In J. Strachey (Ed. and Trans.), *The standard edition of the complete psychological works of Sigmund Freud* (Vol. 14, pp. 243–258). London: Hogarth Press.

Frisch, N. C. (2009). Nursing theory in holistic nursing practice. In B. Dossey & L. Keegan, *Holistic nursing: A handbook for practice* (5th ed., p. 113–123). Sudbury, MA: Jones and Bartlett.

Hess, P. (1990). Loss, grief and dying. In P. Beare & J. L. Meyers (Eds.), *Principles and practices of adult health nursing.* St. Louis, MO: C. V. Mosby.

Holloway, M. (2006). Death the great leveler? Towards a transcultural spirituality of dying and bereavement. *Journal of Clinical Nursing, 15*(7), 833–839.

Kausch, K., & Amer, K. (2007). Self-transcendence and depression among AIDS Memorial Quilt panel makers. *Journal of Psychosocial Nursing Mental Health Services, 45*(6), 44–53.

Kübler-Ross, E. (1969). *On death and dying.* New York: Macmillan.

Kübler-Ross, E. (1975). *Death: The final stage of growth.* Englewood Cliffs, NJ: Prentice Hall.

Kushner, H. S. (1981). *When bad things happen to good people.* New York: Schocken.

Leininger, M. (1978). Transcultural nursing theories and research approaches. In M. Leininger (Ed.), *Transcultural nursing: Concept, theories and practices.* New York: Wiley.

Leininger, M. (1991). *Culture care diversity and universality: A theory of nursing.* New York: National League for Nursing.

Leininger, M. (1998). Special research report: Dominant culture care meanings and practice findings from Leininger's theory. *Journal of Transcultural Nursing, 9*(2), 45–48.

Lindemann, E. (1944). Symptomatology and management of acute grief. *American Journal of Psychiatry, 101*, 141–148.

Love, K. (2008). Interconnectedness in nursing: A concept analysis. *Journal of Holistic Nursing, 26*(4), 255–265.

Neill, J. (2005, October). Health as expanding consciousness: Seven women living with multiple sclerosis or rheumatoid arthritis. *Nursing Science Quarterly, 18*(4), 334–343.

Nightingale, F. (1946). *Notes on nursing* [Facsimile of First Edition, London, 1859]. Philadelphia: Edward Stern & Co.

Nolan, M., & Mock, V. (2004). A conceptual framework for end-of-life care: A reconsideration of factors influencing the integrity of the human person. *Journal of Professional Nursing, 20*(6), 351–360.

Olson, M. (2001). *Healing the dying* (2nd ed.). Albany, NY: Delmar Press.

Palmer, B., Quinn Griffin, M., Reed, P., & Fitzpatrick, J. (2010). Self-transcendence and work engagement in acute care staff registered nurses. *Critical Care Nursing Quarterly, 33*(2), 138–147.

Perry, D. (2004). Self-transcendence: Lonergan's key to integration of nursing theory, research, and practice. *Nursing Philosophy, 5*(1), 67–74.

Persky, G. J., Nelson, J. W., Watson, J., & Bent, K. (2008). Creating a profile of a nurse effective in caring. *Nursing Administration Quarterly, 32*(1), 15–20.

Pipe, T. B. (2008). Illuminating the inner leadership journey by engaging intention and mindfulness as guided by caring theory. *Nursing Administration Quarterly, 32*(2), 117–125.

Puskar, K. R., Brar, L., & Stark, K. H. (2008). Considerations to implement holistic groups with the elderly. *Journal of Holistic Nursing, 26*(3), 212–218.

Reed, P. (1991). Toward a nursing theory of self-transcendence: Deductive reformulation using developmental theories. *Advanced in Nursing Science, 13*(4), 64–77.

Reed, P. (2008). Self transcendence theory. In M. Smith & P. Liehr (Eds.), *Middle range theory for nursing* (p. 105). New York: Springer Publishing Company.

Repede, E. (2008). All that holds: A story of healing. *Journal of Holistic Nursing, 26*(3), 226–232.

Rexroth, R. & Davidbizar, R. (2003). Caring utilizing the Watson theory to transcend culture. *Health Care Manager, 22*, 295–304.

Spence, D., & Smythe, E. (2008). Feeling like a nurse: Re-calling the spirit of nursing. *Journal of Holistic Nursing, 26*(4), 243–252.

Wade, G. H., & Kasper, N. (2006). Nursing students' perceptions of instructor caring: An instrument based on Watson's theory of transpersonal caring. *Journal of Nursing Education, 45*(5), 162–168.

Watson, J. (1988). *Human science and caring*. New Work: National League for Nursing.

Watson, J. (2006a). *Caring science as sacred science*. Philadelphia: F. A. Davis.

Watson, J. (2006b). Caring theory as an ethical guide to administrative and clinical practices. *JONAS Healthc Law Ethics Regulation, 8*(3), 87–93.

Watson, J. (2006c). Caring theory as an ethical guide to administrative and clinical practices. *Nursing Administration Quarterly, 30*(1), 48–55.

Watson, J. (2006d). Walking pilgrimage as caritas action in the world. *Journal of Holistic Nursing, 24*(4), 289–296.

Watson, J. (2009). Caring science and human caring theory: Transforming personal and professional practices of nursing and health care. *Journal Health & Human Services Administration, 31*(4), 466–482.

Watson, J. (2010). Florence Nightingale and the enduring legacy of transpersonal human caring-healing. *Journal of Holistic Nursing, 28*(1), 108.

Waston Caring Institute. Retrieved August 14, 2010, from http://www.watsoncaringscience.org/caring_science/10caritas.htm

Watson Caring Institute, Retrieved August 14, 2010, from http://www.watsoncaringscience.org/caring_science/definitions.html

8 *Letting Go: The Body's Shutdown Process*

To die peacefully, to die with the knowledge that life has had meaning and that one is connected through time and space to others, to
God, and to the universe, is to die well.

—M. Olson and B. Dossey (2009)

*B*ETTY'S STORY   *Betty Riyaja is pretty much alone. Her
husband of 50 years preceded her in death more than four years
ago. Her children, scattered around the country, see her briefly on
their obligatory annual visits. Betty's home is a remote skilled
nursing facility in the upper Midwest. Admitted for dementia about
3 years ago, Betty is now 83.*

*One Sunday night in the middle of winter, Betty has a high fever
and is incontinent; she has worn a diaper for over a year now. The
nurse suspects a urinary tract infection. The ambulance attendants
load her onto a stretcher and take her to the emergency room for
evaluation. By the time all these details are arranged and actualized,
Betty is hemorrhaging. The emergency room doctor does the
preliminary testing and confirms that she is febrile and that her
hemoglobin and hematocrit are dangerously low. Her creatinine
level is at the top of the chart. Further tests diagnose renal failure
with a mass in her lower abdomen. She already has a colostomy due
to a previous tumor 2 years ago. Betty is admitted to the internal
medicine unit. The nurse begins an IV line and adds a unit of packed
cells IV while a general surgery consult is on the way. An aggressive
plan of action commences.*

*Betty slips in and out of consciousness as an all-out war to save
Betty is initiated. A debate between the surgeons begins. Should we
operate now to stent the failing kidney, or should we go in after the
lower pelvic mass? What level of antibiotics should we administer?
The problem is that Betty is too weak to undergo the necessary contrast
material testing to pinpoint the best location to operate. What to do?
In the late night hours the physicians dialogue and ponder their*

options. With no conclusions reached, the bleary-eyed doctors resolve to delay their decision until the next day and go home for a few hours of sleep.

The next day the consultants arrive, making their assessments, logging their clinical notes, and charging the obligatory fees. The nephrologists consider medication to stimulate renal function. The radiologist recommends deferring contrast dye studies for a few days. The internal medicine doctor juggles the hypertension drugs to regulate her blood pressure, while the surgical urologist thinks a stent through the ureter might help. The hospitalist on call writes prescriptions for hypnotics to help her sleep during these interventions while she remains hospitalized. In the meantime the teams continue her IV therapy, respiratory therapy, and intravascular nutrient feedings.

Three days and thousands of Medicare dollars later, Betty overcomes her invasive, inpatient acute care hospital therapies. In the wee hours of an early morning, unwatched and alone in her room, she releases her last painful breath and dies.

REFLECTIONS ON ISSUES OF CONCERN

1. When in the course of medical evaluation can one determine that a person (patient) is in his or her final throes of life?
2. How can we as a society come to accept death as a normal and natural part of life?
3. Is there a way to ease and acknowledge the dying process much as we do the birthing process?
4. How can we protect hospital medical teams from operating out of a sense of fear of litigation?
5. Can we change the laws?
6. Are we willing to change the way we think and to embrace the releasing process, or are we doomed to repeat our old ways of thinking and being?
7. How long will it be until all our health care dollars will be spent prolonging the life of those whose time for release has come?

Consider the old rhyme, "Skipping Rhyme," circa 1894:

> Doctor, doctor, shall I die?
> Yes, my child and so shall I.

The often pain-laden reality is that we are all going to die. The only difference between the dying person and the health care provider is that the dying person in all likelihood will die first (Papadatou, 2009). It could be said that dying, although it will happen to everyone, is the least understood of all the bodily processes because of the overlay of the emotional responses, the spiritual meaning for the person and the family, and the fact that it is the ultimate unknown that must be entered alone. Simply stated, death is a moment in time preceded by dying, which is the end stage of physical life. Dying gives meaning to both life and death (Olson & Dossey, 2009). The process of the body letting go into death is quite possibly the most controversial aspect of the life cycle. Yet within this controversy, the physical process of the body closing down is quite simple and easy to understand.

Fifty years ago people were given palliative care and often died at home surrounded by family and friends. The traditional definition of physical death as the cessation of all bodily functions was easily determined. With the advent of more and more sophisticated revival techniques and life-support treatments, an alternative definition of death was needed, such as "brain death" or "biological death" ("Defining the Moment," 2007). However, in its greatest simplicity, when all the tubes and machines are removed, physical death still remains a cessation of all bodily functions. Death can be seen as both a final shutting down of the body and a particular event with a date, time, and place. Unfortunately, many people do not have the luxury of a peaceful or easy death. The more we recognize this, the better equipped we will be to aid those who suffer at the end of life. Exhibit 8.1 indicates how and why we need to recognize the normal body shutdown process and not push interventions to the point of needless suffering.

The American Geriatrics Society (2007) provides a definitive clue as to when the end of life or dying begins in their *Position Statement on the Care of Dying Patients*: "People are considered to be dying when they are sick with a progressive condition that is expected to end in death and for which there is no treatment that can substantially alter the outcome."

EXHIBIT 8.1   Research Perspective

Face-to-face in-depth qualitative interviews were conducted with 96 terminally ill elders, 15 of whom discussed an event in their dying process that resulted in suffering so great they wished for, or considered, a hastened death. The interviews were conducted on palliative care hospital units, and in outpatient clinics, freestanding hospice facilities, and home hospice settings. Four critical events emerged:

- Perceived insensitive and uncaring communication of a terminal diagnosis
- The experience of unbearable physical pain
- Unacknowledged feelings regarding undergoing chemotherapy or radiation treatment
- The experience of dying in a distressing environment

Respondents discussed physical and/or psychosocial suffering that occurred at these events and the end-of-life care practices that reduced their suffering. The researcher's conclusions were that awareness of events common to the dying process, the potential physical and psychosocial suffering that may arise at these events, and the end-of-life care practices associated with reducing that suffering can lead to health care professionals being able to take a proactive rather than reactive approach to end-of-life care.

From Schroepfer (2007).

The actual dying process usually commences well before the physical death and is a personal journey. Each person's date and time of death are unpredictable. Death, whenever and however it occurs, is likely the single most fearful and least talked-about event in our life. As we age there is the tendency to think more and more about death. Medical personnel will tell you that the actual process of dying has a "final stage," a final physical release. Even if death happens quickly, there is still a final stage, just a very short one. When a disease is involved in the dying process, the individual has time to learn about the impending death and the actual final stage; there is time to prepare for the dying process (Morrow, 2009).

As death approaches, the body begins to shut down in a normal and natural manner. Knowing that physical changes are part of the body letting go is helpful in making end-of-life care decisions and helping loved ones cope with the approach of death. Death, although an inevitable part of the life cycle, is often confusing and frightening for both the dying and their loved ones. Understanding this natural physical process may make it easier to experience (Olson & Dossey, 2009). On the physical plane, the body begins the final process of shutting down, which ends when all the physical systems cease to function. Usually this is an orderly and unromantic progressive series of physical changes. When one is at the end of life and we recognize that this is simply the physical body shutting down, then we can avoid seeing this as a medical emergency requiring invasive interventions. These physical changes are a normal, natural way in which the body prepares itself to stop, and the most appropriate kinds of responses are comfort-enhancing measures (Hospice, 1996).

THE BEGINNING

Currently there seems to be no consensus regarding when dying or the end of life begins (Matzo & Sherman, 2010). Oftentimes a sudden change or decline in health heralds the beginning of the dying process, which can take place several years before actual death. Further, this change or decline is often discernible by body system damage, failure, or subtle change. What seems like a slowing down can in fact be the beginning of the end. This is seen in older people as they become less and less mobile. Their muscle mass, especially in their shoulders, begins to decrease and when hugged they feel frail, although their appearance does not necessarily reflect this fragility. Their diet begins to change, moving more into softer, easier-to-digest foods. Oftentimes these are processed convenience foods. They tend to drink less water, less of everything, as the growing concern is being able to get to the toilet in time. Their day becomes constricted into getting up, dressing, eating breakfast, doing the dishes and perhaps one small activity, and then it is time for lunch, dishes, perhaps a brief rest, and then supper, dishes, and an earlier and earlier bedtime. As this cycle is repeated there is a growing awareness that a lot of things are not being accomplished during the day. It takes all their energy to do the simple tasks of daily living.

There is also a progressive distancing from the world. Although death is the moment a person physically leaves this world, it is preceded by a separating out from the activities of the physical world with a concomitant increasing of intimacy with the vibrational or spiritual world. This distancing can also be seen as an increased attention placed on getting one's affairs in order and planning one's memorial service (Roome, 2008). There seems to be an innate knowing that this physical life is coming to an end, and the preparations to exit are made.

SIGNS OF APPROACHING DEATH

Impending death is heralded by every system of the body and usually begins gradually, often with compensating mechanisms that are not apparent to the untrained eye. See Table 8.1, "Physical Signs of Approaching Death." Some of the signs can be there for years, with more signs and increasing physical deterioration as the years advance. For instance, the skin can be dry and irritated in the 60s, increasing to loose skin from weight loss and paleness in the 70s, and progressing to pressure areas that appear quickly in the 80s, escalating to pressure sores, jaundice, and aversion to the touch of blankets as death is approaching. The signs of impending death can vary greatly from person to person depending on each person's body systems.

TABLE 8.1   Physical Signs of Impending Death

Body System	Signs
Cardiac	Edema of limbs and sacral area
	Possible abdominal swelling
Gastrointestinal	Decreased appetite and weight loss
	Diarrhea and/or constipation
	Mouth sores
	Nausea and/or vomiting
Genitourinary	Bladder spasms and incontinence
	Urinary tract infections
	Urine: foul smelling, concentrated, or cloudy
	Urine retention
Musculoskeletal	Deterioration obvious
	Lethargy, lack of energy, sluggish
	Weakness
	Muscle twitching, limbs especially
Skin	Color: pale, gray, or jaundiced
	Dryness or irritation
	Loose from weight loss
	Pressure sores
	Quickly appearing pressure areas
	Touch aversion, especially for blankets

EXHIBIT 8.2   Neuropsychological Signs of Approaching Death

- Decreasing engagement in outer activities
- Less conversation about family events
- Less empathy with others
- A more inward focus on comfort
- Restlessness

Neuropsychological levels are another indicator of approaching death that varies from person to person. See Exhibit 8.2, "Neuropsychological Signs of Impending Death." In general, there is a turning from interest in the outer world of family and activities to the inner world of comfort, needs, and increasing stillness.

THE LAST DAYS

Gradually, as the signs of impending death advance, it becomes clear that the person has perhaps only 3 to 10 days to live. See Table 8.2, "Physical Changes in the Last Days." The person is physically weak and usually no longer able to get out of bed. The person becomes dependent and cannot participate in any part of his or her self-care. The dying person appears pale and perhaps gaunt, with a touch of jaundice, and requires longer and longer periods of rest. It becomes more difficult for the person to focus and pay attention to things happening in the outer world. As a result poor attention is exhibited, with concentration becoming increasingly disoriented to time and place. See Exhibit 8.3, "Consciousness Changes in the Last Days."

Food is the least of the dying person's concerns, as swallowing becomes more difficult and the gag reflex diminishes. This is the time to have the family come if they have not already arrived, and this is time to have physician write the order for transfer to the *Golden Room.*

Normal Changes in the Last Days

Certainly there are many physical changes that can be observed in the last days that signal the body shutting down and withdrawing its energies into the core. All of them are normal and, once recognized, can assist the health care professional to better help the dying person and his or her family in this process.

TABLE 8.2   Physical Changes in the Last Days

Changes	Verification
Circulation slows	Cold limbs, hands, feet, nose, and ears Diaphoresis Increasing edema, possibly in the lower legs and sacrum Mottling: limbs, nail beds, nose, and ears Skin sensation reduced
Muscle tone reduces	Facial muscles relax Gag reflex decreases gradually Gastrointestinal activity diminishes Sleep time increases Assistance needed with turning in bed/activities of daily living Swallowing problems Urinary/fecal incontinence—relaxed sphincters
Senses diminish	Hearing appears to be the last sense to go Smell declines Taste decreases Touch/sensation lessens Vision fades—often blurry
Vital signs weaken	Blood pressure lowers Breathing: rapid, shallow, slower, irregular Pulse: weak and irregular or rapid

EXHIBIT 8.3   Consciousness Changes in the Last Days

- Hallucinations possible
- Mental function usually declines
- Pain sensation in all probability decreases
- Responsiveness most likely diminished
- Speech: slurring, trailing off, long pauses, phrases
- Varying consciousness: alert to lethargic to comatose
- Visions: perhaps

Appetite

As the digestive system shuts down, food becomes less and less important, and appetite and hunger decrease. Liquids also become less essential. In the last days there comes a time when the person no longer desires to eat or drink. Although small sips might be taken if offered, they are usually not requested. In the words of Kimberly Kimbrough, RN, BSN, a 14-year renal dialysis nurse:

> When they can't feed themselves, feed them.
> When they can't eat, give them fluids.
> When they can't swallow any more, wet their lips.

The body is withdrawing from its need for physical sustenance. There is no longer an appetite and, with that, no hunger pains. The body is closing down all those areas that are no longer needed and conserving the energy expended on these tasks (Morrow, 2009). Eating has both social and symbolic meaning to the person and the family. Remember that taste varies with degrees of illness but stays with us until the end of life. For the person to stop eating in the progression of dying is normal and may not cause undue suffering. Provide food as desired (Olson & Dossey, 2009). For the family these changes can be stressful based on their heritage and background. Food can represent love and often is the central focus of family celebrations. Sometimes the dying person may ask for a favorite food only to be uninterested or unable to eat it when it arrives. Remind the family that this is a normal part of the dying process and their loved one is not starving, not rejecting them, but rather dying. The body is not starving; it is closing down.

Waking and Sleeping Pattern

The person begins to spend less time awake and more time in sleep. Initially the person can be easily aroused from sleep; eventually, the person will seem unconscious and at times be difficult to arouse. This normal change is due in part to changes in the metabolism of the body (Roome, 2008). Increasing sleep may be interpreted by the family as a form of giving up and withdrawing from their love and attention. While health care professionals know this is not true, the family frequently needs guidance to allow the dying person to rest. It is often helpful to suggest that they give their loved one "permission" to rest.

Often the dying person may appear confused as to time, place, and/or the people surrounding the bedside. When this includes close and familiar people, it can be frustrating and heartbreaking. This confusion is due in some part to the metabolic changes (Hospice, 1996). At this stage dreams and visions of God and paradise are common. Although the person becomes more and more unresponsive, he or she can still hear. It is important to keep talking with him or her, touching and caring. Sometimes, as death approaches a person may have a final burst of wakefulness and clarity in which he or she talks to those present or acknowledges them in some way. This is usually short-lived (Roome, 2008).

Body Systems

The digestion and elimination systems are among the first to close down. Oftentimes there is a profuse amount of elimination as the body prepares for death and the sphincter muscles relax. As the synaptic gaps occasionally misfire in shutting down, there is muscle twitching in the arms, hands, and legs. When this happens in the hands, it can be misinterpreted as the dying person trying to communicate with someone who is holding his or her hand. Swelling in the extremities or lungs results if the heart is struggling to pump properly. Shaking is a common side effect of the body systems shutting down. Holding a person close and rocking gently is often the best treatment for the person and for those in attendance (Hospice, 1996).

Breathing

With approaching death, the breath rate begins to slow drastically, with breaths becoming farther and farther apart. Normally, death is not imminent while the breathing remains quiet and gentle. The person may have gurgling sounds coming from his or her chest as though marbles were rolling around inside; this is commonly known as the "death rattle." These sounds may become very loud. This normal change is due to the decrease of fluid intake and an inability to cough up normal secretions. Suctioning sometimes increases the secretions and may cause sharp discomfort (Hospice, 1996).

The normal breathing pattern often changes with the start of a different breathing rate. One pattern often seen consists of breathing irregularly, such as shallow breaths with periods of no breathing varying from 5 to 30 seconds. This is called Cheyne–Stokes breathing. Another pattern consists of periods of rapid, shallow, pant-like breathing. These patterns are very common and indicate decrease in circulation in the internal organs (Hospice, 1996).

With approaching death breathing often becomes labored, with a gasping for air. This is called "fish-out-of-water" breathing. This is an exaggerated gulping motion giving the appearance of trying to get one more breath (Parsons, 2007). These breaths then slow, coming further and further apart until the final exhalation. The moment of actual physical death has no pain; it is a reflex last exhalation (Olson & Dossey, 2009).

Circulation, Skin, and Blood Pressure

During the last few days the blood pressure and pulse can become erratic, with no regular pattern. The blood pressure begins to become more erratic as heart rate and pumping gradually lessen in frequency, volume, and intensity. Sometimes this causes emotional side effects, such as outbursts of anger and grief. The family needs to be reminded that these are side effects and not to be taken personally (Roome, 2008). The regulation of body temperature begins to falter, and the extremities can feel very cold one minute and another minute warm. Mottled skin becomes apparent around the mouth, nose, and extremities. Mottled skin on dependent body parts such as buttocks or the back appears as bruising as the person is turned over or onto one side. Skin color changes range from clammy or flushed to a gray/blue color. The circulation is slowly being withdrawn from the outer limbs and being concentrated in the major internal organs (Morrow, 2009).

Nutrition and Hydration

As the body continues to shut down there is less and less need for calories and fluids. Rather than seeking energy to sustain itself and live, the body is letting go and preparing to stop all functions. This is an autoregulatory function involving neither pain nor suffering. The person is not thirsty, although a dry mouth might be experienced that can be comforted with a moist cloth applied to the lips. When we are conscious that this occurrence is a normal part of the shutdown and release process there are less guilt and desire to insist that our loved one drink and/or to force fluids on the person during this dying process. It is often thought that in the last hours of life the dehydration causes no suffering but rather stimulates the release of endorphins and anesthetic compounds, which give the person a sense of well-being.

Intravenous fluids are often considered at this point in time or are already in place. While these fluids can be supportive for some symptoms, the body can become overloaded because it is shutting down; this can cause increasing shortness of breath and possible painful edema. Instead, mouth care with swabs and ice chips can help prevent dryness and be comforting.

Restlessness and Agitation

The person may make restless and repetitive motions such as pulling at bed linens or clothing. This often happens and is due in part to the decrease in oxygen circulation to the brain and to metabolism changes. There is no pain or feeling of distress here. It is not necessary to interfere with or try to restrain such motions (Hospice, 1996). Agitation is often an indication of a simple, treatable cause such as urinary retention or uncontrolled pain that can be easily remedied.

Senses

All the senses change as the body slowly shuts down. For smell there is a decrease in awareness of aromas or the smell of food, though for awhile odors can cause nausea and an unsettled stomach. The person loses interest in and stops enjoying the taste of food. As death approaches the eyes may remain open with a glassy stare that indicates a withdrawal of sensory perception from the external environment. Sometimes the dying reach their hands upward. Death generally occurs within hours after the eyes become glassy and fixed. The sense of hearing is often sharp to the end of physical life. Hearing appears to be the last sense to leave (Olson & Dossey, 2009).

Urine and/or Bowel Changes

As the muscles of the internal organs begin to relax, the dying person may become incontinent and experience diarrhea. The urine output normally decreases, becoming concentrated and tea colored from decreased fluid intake and decreasing circulation through the kidneys.

IMMINENT DEATH

Within hours or sometimes minutes of dying, the body begins its final shutdown of all systems. See Exhibit 8.4, "Signs of Imminent Death." Most noticeably the pupils become dilated and fixed, with the pulse weaker yet faster and the blood pressure lowering. The dying person is still, with no body movements, and usually has minimal if any words

EXHIBIT 8.4   Signs of Imminent Death

- Blood pressure continues to drop
- Cheyne–Stokes respirations occur
- Death rattle is heard
- Movement ceases
- Pulse weakens and becomes faster
- Pupils are dilated and fixed
- Speech is minimal or absent

to say. Cheyne–Stokes respirations have longer and longer pauses, and a "death rattle" is often heard. There is no pain, simply a closing down of all body functions.

A MOMENT IN TIME: DEATH

Death is an amazing transition. One minute the dying person is alive, though minimally, and the next, there is no "life" in the body. The life is gone, and there is only a physical body, which rapidly begins to decompose. Although we may anticipate it, we can never be prepared for the moment of physical death. It is a final closure that is irreversible for just about everyone. Clinical death has six components. Exhibit 8.5, "Clinical Death," lists these six events.

Briefly stated, breathing ceases, the eyes no longer respond to light, the pulse stops, reflexes are nonresponsive, external stimuli provoke no response, and the muscles no longer move. What you may observe is tight brow muscles becoming relaxed and a peace in the face (Olson & Dossey, 2009).

EXHIBIT 8.5   Clinical Death

- Breathing—none
- External stimuli—no response
- Eyes—no response
- Muscle movement—none
- Pulse—none
- Reflexes—none

Words of Wisdom

"The best plan for preparing for a good death begins years before death occurs. Learn to practice the art of letting go in everyday matters both great and small. Let go of perceived psychological hurts. Move with and into physical pain until the source of it abates. Accept a spiritual belief system. Release unused or unneeded items in your life. Give away things in your personal environment that no longer call to you, i.e., jewelry that you haven't worn in years, items from your storage locker or attic, or what has accumulated as clutter in your personal space. Practice the art of letting go every day."

L. Keegan (personal communication, 2010).

SUMMARY

The picture of death looks something like this physically:

- The heart stops beating.
- Breathing stops.
- The body color becomes pale.
- The body cools.
- Muscles relax.
- Urine and stool may be released.
- The eyes may remain open.
- The jaw can fall open.
- Trickling of internal fluids may be heard. (Michigan State, 2001)

Reflect for a moment on how you would feel if your loved one, or even you yourself, died alone in an intensive care unit or in a nursing home. *The Golden Room* personnel can offer care, trust, compassion, acceptance, and loving support to journey through the final chapter of one's life with dignity. The family memories of how a loved one died will live on in them. Will those memories be painful or full of love and appreciation of a gentle death surrounded by loved ones?

No one knows the exact time or place of his or her death. In the final days the body's letting go increases in intensity, affecting all organs and systems. Nothing is left unaffected. Once understood, physical death no longer needs to be feared but rather can once again be seen as a natural part of the life cycle. Every one of us will experience death, no exceptions.

REFERENCES

American Geriatrics Society. (2007). *Position statement on the care of dying patients* [Electronic version]. Retrieved May 17, 2010, from http://www.americangeriatrics.org/products/positionpapers/careofd.shtml

Defining the moment of death. (2007). *Dear Death.* Retrieved February 16, 2010, from http://www.deardeath.com/physical_death.html

Hospice. (1996). *Preparing for approaching death.* Florida: North Central Florida Hospice. Accessed February 16, 2009, from http://www.hospicenet.org/html/preparing_for.html

Matzo, M., & Sherman, D. (Eds.). (2010). *Palliative care nursing: Quality care to the end of life* (3rd ed.). New York: Springer Publishing Company.

Michigan State University. (2001). *Completing a life: Signs of death.* Accessed February 17, 2010, from http://www.commtechlab.msu.edu/sites/completingalife/audioon/tc/signs_death.html

Morrow, A. (2009). *The journey towards death: Recognizing the dying process.* Retrieved May 18, 2010, from http://dying.about.com/od/thedyingprocess/a/process.htm

Olson, M., & Dossey, B. (2009). Dying in peace. In B. Dossey & L. Keegan, *Holistic nursing: A handbook for practice* (5th ed., pp. 393–414). Sudbury, MA: Jones and Bartlett.

Papadatou, D. (2009). *In the face of death.* New York: Springer Publishing Company.

Parsons, P. (2007). Language of the butterfly. In C. Drick (Ed.), *Mother stories: Through our mothers' death and dying* (pp. 213–232). Charleston, SC: BookSurge.

Roome, D. (2008). Physical changes before death: How the body shuts down as death approaches. *Suite101.com.* Retrieved May 18, 2010, from http://cancer.suite101.com/article.cfm/physical_changes_before_death

Schroepfer, T. A. (2007). Critical events in the dying process: The potential for physical and psychosocial suffering. *Journal of Palliative Medicine, 10*(1), 136–147.

9 Changing the Consciousness around Death and Dying

Matter can be neither created nor destroyed, but only changed in form.

—First law of physics

MOM'S STORY   *The day after Christmas, Mom had a mild transient ischemic attack (TIA). She completely recovered and had a very engaged day with us, laughing, relaxing, working on her crossword puzzles, and reading. When asked if she wanted to discuss her TIA, she smiled and said, "No thank you. I am very aware of what happened since many of my friends have experienced them." She went on laughingly, "Well, my brain is getting a little less confused, and it simply is just what happened. Thank heavens I'm now here, alert, talking, walking, and moving!"*

There was a palpable presence that radiated from Mom all day that was extraordinary. With an "engaged watching," Mom seemed to track all of us in our activities or conversations in a different way. My sister and I commented on this to her. Mom gave us her adorable, wide smile in which her eyes would always disappear. The rest of the day she looked at us as if she knew that her time with us was coming to an end. This was very possible because it is not unusual for a stroke to follow a TIA. But most of all there seemed to be an inner wisdom coming forth.

That evening Mom was very tired and went to bed at 10:30 p.m. My sister, sensing something was wrong since Mom didn't kiss us goodnight, went to her room and found her confused. My husband, Larry, and I went to her bedroom. Her last words to us were "take me home." We told her that she was at home and that if by chance she saw another place called home she should feel free to go there. Because she was confused, I told Larry that I was going to stay with her until she went back to sleep, and I climbed into her bed. I had done this so many times, either to chat or watch a television movie with her. I was aware that this could be my last time to be with her and felt a deep sense of this being a sacred space and time.

Since Mom was resting on her back, I lay on my right side and rested my hand on the center of her chest; she immediately placed both her hands on mine. I gently turned my hand and grasped hers. We both drifted to sleep. Mom had a massive stroke at 2:05 a.m. on December 27. She became diaphoretic, which woke me up. I saw that Mom's eyes were deviated to one side and that she was unresponsive. I knew that the most important thing was just to be with her in these precious moments. I never imagined that I would be with her in this time between two worlds. This experience of "being with" remains beyond words. My tears were joyful, and I was conscious of releasing her in this physical life form. Certainly my meditation practice of releasing attachment to the physical body had become part of my beingness.

About 30 minutes later, Larry awoke and came to Mom's room to check on us. Since Mom had signed her living will, we honored her wishes and provided comfort care, love, and prayers in her home for the next two days. We intuitively knew that this was the right thing to do. The knowingness that was coming forward was that this was a sacred journey with Mom.

Although she was unresponsive, Mom's blood pressure and heartbeat were strong. Hospice was called, and we sat with her, reading her favorite Bible verses and simply being present. Mom made her transition with elegance, grace, and gentleness on December 30 at 2:58 a.m. (adapted from B. Dossey, 2008)

REFLECTIONS ON ISSUES OF CONCERN

1. Engaged watching is common in dying persons, most often for those who are awake, aware, and accepting of what is happening. Is it possible for this to become the norm rather than the exception? Could engaged watching become a sign of approaching death rather than a phenomenon rarely seen? What would it take?

2. The experience of "being with" someone who is between two worlds is invaluable. How can we make this a common, acceptable experience? Would the *Golden Room* assist those who are reticent to stay and experience this sacred time?

3. Intuitively knowing the right thing to do is not commonly expressed in a clinical situation. As we become more comfortable with death as a natural part of life, how do you see this changing?
4. What aspect of change theory most clearly resonates with the dying process?
5. What would it take to make death a more comfortable topic for friends and loved ones to talk about? How comfortable are you and your family in talking about and planning for this finality?
6. There are five poignant inner gifts of death and dying: goodness, compassion, peace, dignity, and release. Which among these are you least comfortable with? How will you go about changing your level of comfort?

CHANGING CONSCIOUSNESS

Changing the consciousness around death and dying to one of acceptance and reverence of this, the second of the two most important events in physical life, the first being birth, is perhaps the most exciting and most challenging aspect of implementing the *Golden Room* in different settings. Physical change based on concrete facts and information can be readily dealt with in a logical and sequential process. Changing consciousness, however, becomes challenging because it deals with the more amorphous areas of history, emotions, customs, peer pressure, and much more. Thus it is important to look at change theory to begin to understand the process and ways to implement change for both society in general and the health care system in particular.

Change Theory

An overview of Lewin's change theory is presented first. This is probably one of the most powerful models of the change process in humans and human systems (Schein, 2002). It further clarifies and assists our understanding of the process involved in changing the consciousness around death and dying. The more specific arena of change theory adapted to nursing and nursing care is then addressed.

Planned change was first introduced by Kurt Lewin in 1951 as a 3-step change model consisting of unfreezing, change, and refreezing; it is outlined in Table 9.1. This model considers that present concepts and ideas are discarded, and new concepts and ideas are put in their place. In stage 1 the unfreezing of the present situation is begun by increasing the motivational sources and decreasing the preventive forces, then blending the two as the unfreezing continues. Motivation and readiness are the two areas of action that assist this unfreezing. In stage 2, once the desire to change and enough dissatisfaction are present, the specific change needed is identified. Finally, in stage 3, the refreezing occurs as the new concepts and ideas and the corresponding new behaviors become customary, resulting in a new identity, a new self-concept, and new levels of communicating with others (Wirth, 2004).

Change Theory in Nursing and Nursing Care

In their dual role as caregivers and organization "keepers," nurses may already have the key to creating a culture of engagement. Both theory and theory change are necessary as one looks at end-of-life care. The characteristics and benefits of engaging work environments are captured in nursing professional practice models, as evidenced by a quarter century of research on magnet hospitals and professional practice. An inflection point, providing an opportunity for transformational change in the nursing work environment, may be generated by a critical need for nurses and a call for redesign of the health care delivery system (Fasoli, 2010). One such theory of system redesign is Rizzo Parse's humanbecoming leading-following model, which can be used by nurses practicing within most nursing care settings (Doucet & Maillard-

TABLE 9.1   Lewin's 3-Step Change Model

Steps	Process/Actions
1. Unfreeze present behavior/ situation	Increase motivating forces
	Decrease preventive forces
	Merge the two methods
2. Change	View status quo as not beneficial
	Promote fresh viewpoint
	Work collectively
	Connect viewpoint to respected, influential leaders supporting change
3. Refreezing	Integrate new traditions and values

Schein, E. (2002). *Kurt Lewin's change theory in the field and in the classroom: Notes toward a model of managed learning.* Retrieved February 23, 2010, from http://www.a2zpsychology.com/articles/kurt_lewin's_change_theory.htm

Strüby, 2009). The humanbecoming leading-following model challenges the traditional notion of leadership. The model is a guide to living leading-following with a focus on human dignity and freedom where power is with the constituents of situations (Rizzo Parse, 2008). The humanbecoming family model offers an alternative view of family. The essences, paradoxes, and processes offer a unique way of envisioning family (Parse, 2009). Another model, self-determination theory, promotes healthy behavior change in clients. When nurses act in ways that support clients' innate needs for autonomy, competence, and relatedness, clients may be more successful at internalizing self-regulation and more inclined to adopt and maintain lifelong behavioral changes (Johnson, 2007). These and other change theories may be applied to rethinking how we care for the terminally ill.

CHANGING OUR CONSCIOUSNESS AROUND DEATH AND DYING

It could be said that we enter this physical world with the help of specially trained physicians, nurses, and auxiliary personnel; a specialized room and equipment; and active family participation, and get out of this physical world the best way that we can. Death, although inevitable, is a topic seldom talked about in families until it is at our doorstep, and then it is discussed in hushed tones, often with great anguish.

For the individual approaching death it is even more difficult. When those dying approach their families wanting to talk about death and dying, they are usually brushed off, encouraged to look at the positive side, or reassured that all is well. Most dying persons learn to play the "elephant on the table" game that families unknowingly have created. In this game everyone knows what is happening yet no one speaks about it or acknowledges it to the other people present except perhaps in random hushed moments of emotional release. As a result, the elephant grows larger and larger, and as it turns or moves on the table, everyone experiences increasing inner turmoil but no one acknowledges it openly. An essential condition for providing optimal care to cancer patients, for example, is a thorough understanding of these patients' worries and needs. Exhibit 9.1 shows how essential it is to be conscious of patients' concerns and worries.

Although physical death is seen as the final life experience, we are in truth dying each day. Each morning when we awake we are beginning a new day different from the day before. Although many things

EXHIBIT 9.1   Research Perspective

A Dutch study assessed and compared the perceptions of health care providers and patients about the impact of cancer and chemotherapy. The research group included breast cancer survivors ($n = 80$), oncology nurses ($n = 41$), and physicians with oncology experience ($n = 49$) who completed a psychophysical scale with items tapping both the physical and psychosocial effects of cancer and chemotherapy. The results demonstrated that the following five issues ranked highest among patients: fear of metastases, fatigue, consciousness of one's own vulnerability, hair loss, and nausea. There was a strong correspondence between the ratings of nurses and physicians, as both groups grossly overestimated and underestimated various issues. For example, nurses greatly overestimated the effects on relationships with partners and children, while physicians mostly underestimated hair loss. It was not surprising to discover a considerable discrepancy between patients' and medical professionals' perceptions on various issues. Based on this clinicians can realize that the observed lack of correspondence between patients and health care providers may result in inappropriate provision of attention and health care. Methods have to be developed to assess easily the main needs and worries of individual patients, which is essential to be able to provide optimal care.

From Mulders, Vingerhoets, and Breed (2008).

appear to be the same, it is really a totally different experience. Our mind tells us that this day is the same as the previous day because we are doing similar things. However, the reality is that this day is completely different, this moment is completely different, a one-of-a-kind, never-to-be-repeated existence. Although we may try to bring back the experience again and again, it can never be exactly repeated. Life continually moves forward, not backward. What happened yesterday is now a memory, and try as we might we cannot relive a memory exactly as it happened. It simply is not possible.

Consider your breath. During the day we breathe thousands of times, and each breath, though similar, is different—different intensity, different depth, different situation; pausing, holding, sighing; changing while talking, listening, thinking, moving. The list can go on and on.

Each breath is specific and unique to that moment. And what happens at the end of the breath? We go on to the next breath without giving the former breath another thought. We, in fact, die to the previous breath and turn to the next breath repeatedly, again and again. Have you ever thought, "Well, my best breath was about 5 years ago . . . in the summer. June, no July the 15th . . . yes the 15th . . . It was in the afternoon just after swimming . . . 2:30, no 2:34 p.m." No, we simply take our breath for granted unless we are having difficulty breathing. Each day we are dying thousands of times to our breath, to the moment, and turning to the next breath, the next moment without a thought of holding on to the last moment. Our life is composed of millions of tiny deaths each day, and yet we fear our or a loved one's last breath.

As we contemplate the tiny deaths that occur each day, a realization begins to emerge. Death is a normal part of physical life, both the large and small daily deaths and the larger, end-of-life death. Physical life begins with birth, moves through life experiences, and ends with death. Life is a continuous process of physical, mental, and emotional changing, and we can experience life only in the present moment. This is the only moment we have. This moment appears to change yet underneath it life is always the same; however, the form that it takes changes.

When life is simplified to these simple terms, death begins to take on a new perspective. Death is not something to be feared or hushed away. It really is okay to die. And just as we talk about other events in our life, it is okay to talk about death. The scary part that we feel is all the unconscious emotions coming up based on past unintegrated feelings about old losses in our life that we could not do anything about. The positive part is that acknowledging the feelings surrounding the impending death assists in resolving the past emotions.

When we acknowledge the feelings we are having—that we are feeling scared, abandoned, alone, unsupported, failing, and so on—we are able to bring the light of consciousness to the situation. In doing so we begin to realize that it is allright to have these feelings, that they are part of the experience. This makes the feelings neither good nor bad, simply what we are experiencing.

As we recognize the feelings for what they are, memories, we no longer have to be unconsciously controlled by them. These memories are not real. They are the past and we are living in the present. We live in this moment. As we let go of the shackles of unconscious feelings, we begin to realize just how much they have been preventing us from being alive and responding in this moment to what is actually

Words of Wisdom

"The influence of religious beliefs and practices at the end of life is underinvestigated. Given nursing's advocacy role and the intimate and personal nature of the dimensions of religiosity and the end of life, exploring the multidimensional interplay of religiosity and end-of-life care is a significant aspect of the nurse-patient relationship and must be better understood. The question that must be faced is whether nurses' own belief systems impinge on or influence patient care, especially for patients who are at the end of life. When nurses understand their own beliefs and respect the religious practices and needs of patients and their families, it deepens the humanistic dimensions of the nurse-patient relationship."

From Bjarnason (2009, p. 517).

happening. We become more understanding and accepting of ourselves and others. We begin to show up in our life and what we are experiencing. We begin to discover the inner gifts of goodness, compassion, peace, dignity, and release. We begin to realize the importance of a place for death with dignity, a place called the *Golden Room*.

INNER GIFTS

There are many inner gifts that begin to show up in our life as we more consciously pay attention to our life and how it is flowing. Five gifts are poignant in the context of death and dying. They are detailed in Exhibit 9.2. Each represents an important attribute underlying a consciousness that moves us beyond the fear and numbness of the finality of physical death. This shift in consciousness is fundamental not only to transcend death but also to be truly alive in our present life in this moment. Without this shift in consciousness we remain stuck in our past experiences and can learn nothing more. This oftentimes means living a life of quiet desperation rather than enjoying the fullness of life that our creator intended for us.

Because of the innateness of these gifts, no research can actually measure them or directly demonstrate or capture them for our mind to understand. Instead, these gifts are inner gifts of feelings that in and

EXHIBIT 9.2   Five Inner Gifts of the End of Life

- Goodness
- Compassion
- Peace
- Dignity
- Release

of themselves are more amorphous. For each of us these gifts take on different meanings such that attempting to define them would mean putting them in a box and limiting and often stopping the self-discovery on our personal journey through life. Rather than leading our life based on someone else's definition and ideas, what if we can discover for ourselves the deeper meaning, the significance of these gifts in our lives?

Goodness

Goodness is a word we do not hear very often these days; it describes a quality of decency, kindness, honesty, integrity, and even righteousness, which are simple yet profound qualities that emerge through present-moment living. For health care providers it is about offering care in a kind and gentle manner that neither takes shortcuts nor is influenced by extraneous circumstances such as the health care provider's personal life and opinions. It is about being there in the moment to assist this person and family to move into solutions. It is about taking the time to be fully present for whatever is needed at this moment, whether it is moistening the dying person's lips or rubbing the shoulders of a family member tired from a long night of vigilant watching and waiting. It is about the kindness and decency of caring for someone in an irreversible, inevitable situation.

For the family, goodness is about being with mother, father, sibling, or child and not shying away from personal feelings, being open and honest; no elephant on the table here. Instead, goodness is sharing from the heart and allowing the dying one to also share and be open as to what he or she is feeling and experiencing. So often the feelings of the dying person and the family are similar; their shared insights assist in mutual clarity and understanding. It is often both the tears of sadness and the shared laughter in the end of life that survivors remember.

For the dying person, goodness is about the freedom to express himself or herself and the time to drink in all the kindness and gifts of being in this moment surrounded by people, family and caregivers, who are also in this moment. And being here, at the time between two worlds, the dying person can feel safe knowing that what is physically needed is being taken care of and all he or she has to do is to allow this natural process to gently and easily take place. He or she can relax into this moment of being. Goodness becomes a worthy thing to do and evolves naturally as we live in the present moment and discover what each moment offers to us as we respond from awareness rather than from fear.

Compassion

Compassion is about just that, "come-pass-on," which is to pass on the gentle concern, consideration, and care that assist the dying person in experiencing as much as possible the gentle death that we all hope for. Compassion speaks to being there in empathy, feeling deeply, and acknowledging our feelings to ourselves and moving deeper into these feelings and discovering the release in the center of them. This is moving beyond the given to being with the person in consciousness and becoming so blended that oftentimes no words are needed, as things are just known and accepted.

Compassion arises from a deep inner knowing that, beyond the appearance, beyond the final outcome, somehow, in some way, things are just as they are supposed to be and death and dying are simply another phase in the physical life cycle. The gentleness that is expressed to the dying person and the family is beyond explanation. It is like a transmission of unconditional love passing through the sense of touch, the sound of the voice, the look in the eyes. It is the light and love of God coming through.

Peace

The peace often associated with death is the "peace that passes all understanding." This is the deep inner peace that our soul desires to pass gently into the next world. This peace has often been described as a quiet calm, an inner stillness, and comfortable silence that feels as if everything in one's life and in the universe is in harmony. It reflects a deep connectedness to all that is and all that ever will be.

This is the "felt" peace that is inside us even in the midst of chaos or pain on the outside. It is a felt peace regardless of the appearance or situation. It is the peace that comes from knowing that everything really is moving along just as it needs to even though our human mind cannot control, change, or even comprehend it. This peace is reflective of being in the present moment, of living in the present moment and accepting life on its terms. And accepting life on its terms means that we cannot always control what happens in our life. What we can control is the quality with which we move through our life. This peace is the deepest depth of the Serenity Prayer, "God, grant me the serenity to accept the things I cannot change; courage to change the things I can; and wisdom to know the difference."

Dignity

Dignity is the recognition of each person as worthy of respect and gentleness, with an acceptance of death as a natural part of life. As we allow ourselves to move more and more in the present moment, we begin to discover a dignity, a reverence for all of life. We begin to respect each other and have a humble pride with respect and poise even toward ourselves.

Death is a life-changing experience for all involved. A sacred dignity becomes evident as we allow ourselves to be in the moment, to feel our feelings in the moment, and allow others to feel their feelings without shame or guilt. Death with dignity is giving respect and esteem to both the dying person and the process of death. There is a mystery here that we can only guess and speculate about. But that mystery does not have to be shunned, but rather with dignity we can honor and respect the sacredness of what is occurring.

In a larger sense as nurses we have made a commitment to caring for people and assisting them through changing health situations. Caring for another person is intimate, sacred work. We always have a choice as to how we work with people. We can grin and grind through each step steeped in our own worries and concerns about how much we have to do, with little respect and gentleness for ourselves and this sacred work that we are doing. Or we can be in this moment with poise and deep awareness of the reverence for life and these last moments of it. As we have dignity in ourselves, we discover that the gentle dignity of others and their situations naturally emerges.

Release

Release becomes evident as we allow the natural order of death and dying to flow gently and easily without hindering it by hopeless attempts to detain the inevitable. Throughout life many consciously living people strive for and have learned again and again to let go of material things easily and gently. Some have much practice with this: letting go of clothes that no longer fit, letting go of a job, letting go of a relationship, moving to a new home or new location, or graduating from school. Releasing is sometimes voluntary. Sometimes it is forced on us through being fired from a job, getting a divorce, dropping a prized family heirloom that breaks, or being robbed. It is not the releasing that is the challenge but rather the emotion that goes along with it. Death is a fact. The fact is not the challenge. The emotion that goes along with death is the challenge.

As we live more and more in the present moment and acknowledge our feelings as they arise and feel them with the little daily things, then when the big things come along, we are better able to feel the emotion, acknowledge the emotion, and allow the emotion to be without trying to stuff it or change it. Then the releasing can occur with greater ease. There is a natural cycle, an order to this thing we call life. Releasing, letting go of the physical, is a natural part of the life cycle.

Gratitude

Coming full cycle, with these end-of-life inner gifts, one begins to feel a sense of deep gratitude. This occurs for the caregiver, the family, and the dying person and comes in the form of a deep knowing that all is well. Everything is being taken care of, and this feeling assists in the gentle release from this physical world. All may feel the sacred honor of being with this person at this time of being between two worlds. This is the deep gratitude for life, for the journey, for being that is beyond words. Exhibit 9.3 gives an example of a healing end-of-life ritual.

THE IMPORTANCE OF A PLACE
FOR DEATH WITH DIGNITY

Beginning to live life on its terms and showing up in our life here in the present moment, we begin to experience a sacredness of all life and the life cycle. We begin to realize that every living thing has a time to

EXHIBIT 9.3   Point of View

R ituals at End of Life
      Presence is what serves us in healing the wounds of loss
and grief. I waited until 7:00 a.m. to call the family to tell them about
Mom becoming unresponsive. Together, my sister and I made a
"to do" list and set in motion immediate tasks and people to contact. Mom's doctor placed her on hospice; within a few hours the
hospice nurse had helped us create the flow of comfort-care procedures and medication for Mom. The family engaged in healing
rituals such as bathing Mom, reading her favorite Bible verses,
and sitting quietly with her. This was a time of moving with intention in slow motion; there was no rushing. We made sure we
included Mom's two caregivers and her young sisters who had
attended her since late September. Throughout the day we sat
with Mom, either together or alone for extended periods. For all
of us to be present in these last hours was utterly sacred. Beyond
words we could feel this sacredness deepen as the veil between
the physical world and the spiritual world became very thin.
      Several hours prior to her death, we gave Mom a final bath,
washed and set her hair, painted her nails with pale, golden polish,
and placed her favorite golden lipstick on her, and then dressed
her in a beige gown. It was an honoring of her physical body and
preparation for the soul's journey home. All of my life's work in
holistic nursing and compassionate care of the dying seemed to
be for this moment.

Adapted from Dossey (2008).

be born, a time to grow and flourish, a time to mature, and a time to
die. Everything progresses through this cycle. No one is immune. As
we begin to hold all life as sacred, we begin to desire every moment
of this precious existence to be at the very highest and best level for
ourselves and others.

As we view our life we realize that many parts of it are already at this
level. Many other parts of our life are not. As we experience the death
and dying of loved ones, we realize that we want the very best, the
most comfortable, and the most loving circumstance for them. As caregivers we begin to realize that each life is sacred, each passing an honor
to attend. Each death is unique, never to be duplicated or repeated.

As we accept the natural cycle of life, we especially desire an easy passage through death without all the tubes, invasive medical interventions, IVs, and monitors. With this change of consciousness we realize that death is not an ending but really is a transition to something else. *Matter can neither be created nor destroyed, only changed in form.* We realize that this is a sacred passage, a time of honoring, a time for goodness, a time for compassion, a time for peace, dignity, and most of all gentle release.

We realize that our thinking about death needs to shift into a place of growing ease and ability to look at the finality of life and not be scared into avoiding talking about or planning for it. We realize that having a place for death with dignity is necessary not just for ourselves but for everyone who desires it. *The Golden Room* can provide a place for this often-welcomed rite of passage. It is time to create a place for ourselves, our loved ones, and others who desire it.

All of us face physical death.

This is a fact.

There are no exceptions.

SUMMARY

In order for anything to manifest on this physical plane it is first created in thought. With the realization in thought the expression in form then appears. When we understand this basic principle of life it becomes apparent that it is time for the consciousness around death and dying to change. This is seen with the writing of this book. Concomitant with this change in consciousness, the next step in death with dignity for everyone is the *Golden Room*.

REFERENCES

Bjarnason, D. (2009). Nursing, religiosity, and end-of-life care: Interconnections and implications. *Nursing Clinics of North America, 44*(4), 517–525.

Dossey, B. (2008). She is now wherever we are. In C.A. Drick (Ed.), *Mother stories: Through our mothers' death and dying* (pp. 25–36). North Carolina: BookSurge.

Doucet, T., & Maillard-Strüby, F. (2009). The humanbecoming leading-following model in practice. *Nursing Science Quarterly, 22*(4), 333–338.

Fasoli, D. (2010). The culture of nursing engagement: A historical perspective. *Nursing Administration Quarterly, 34*(1), 18–29.

Johnson, V. (2007). Promoting behavior change: Making healthy choices in wellness and healing choices in illness—Use of self-determination theory in nursing practice. *Nursing Clinicals of North America, 42*(2), 229–241.

Mulders, M., Vingerhoets, A., & Breed, W. (2008). The impact of cancer and chemotherapy: Perceptual similarities and differences between cancer patients, nurses and physicians. *European Journal of Oncology Nursing: The Official Journal of the European Oncology Nursing Society, 12*(2), 97–102.

Parse, R. (2009). The humanbecoming family model. *Nursing Science Quarterly, 22*(4), 305–309.

Parse, R. (2008). The humanbecoming leading-following model. *Nursing Science Quarterly, 21*(4), 369–375.

Schein, E. (2002). *Kurt Lewin's change theory in the field and in the classroom: Notes toward a model of managed learning.* Retrieved February 23, 2010, from http://www.a2zpsychology.com/articles/kurt_lewin's_change_theory.htm

Wirth, R. (2004). *Lewin/Schein's change theory.* Retrieved February 18, 2010, from http://www.entarga.com/orgchange/lewinschein.pdf

10 Spiritual Perspectives

Do you have the patience to wait until the mud settles and the water clears?

—Lao-Tzu

*B*ERTHA'S STORY   *At 93 years young Bertha was the picture of health, living in her own home, active in her church community, cooking for her grandchildren, great-grandchildren, and great-great-grandchildren as well as enjoying her gardening. One morning after her daily routine of yoga, breathing exercises, meditation, and an affirmative reading for the day, she began to feel a little lightheaded. A good breakfast helped some, but she continued to feel slightly dizzy so she called her general practitioner, who suggested she come in for a quick checkup.*

Sitting in his office the next week she was surprised to find that her 72-year-old physician, Tom, had taken on a 31-year-old partner, Dr. Frank. Tom planned to retire at the end of the year. She briefly saw Tom as he introduced her to Dr. Frank. Dr. Frank was gentle but insisted on a complete physical "to get to know her." Dr. Frank listened to her carotid arteries, then insisted on an angiogram immediately. Bertha responded that Tom had always listened to "her neck" over the years and was watching it. She asked why Dr. Frank was now insisting on a test.

Reluctantly she agreed, although on leaving she said to him in her quiet, gentle way, "I've led a good life and I'm 93. I'm really fine if it's my time." Dr. Frank answered her by saying the test was only diagnostic and not to worry. He wanted to get a full picture of her health. Bertha immediately went home and called her minister for prayer, asking for healing and for God's will to be done. The next day she called and scheduled the angiogram. The first opening was in a month.

In the ensuing weeks Bertha had very infrequent times of lightheadedness; at these times she would sit down or lie down and take a healthy dose of prayer. She thought to put a note on her desk with the location of her will and her daughters' telephone numbers.

She decided not to alarm her children as Dr. Frank said this was nothing, just needed to get a full picture of her health.

On the morning of the angiogram Bertha did her normal routine and then drove herself to the hospital. Things were strange and a little intimidating, so rushed and hurried, but she adjusted, knowing this was only a test and she could return home as soon as this was done. During the procedure she endured the positioning, the coolness of the room, and people talking over her and waited patiently for it all to be over. The doctor did not seem pleased with the results and left the room. When he returned he said that they needed to immediately admit Bertha as her carotids were 95% and 100% blocked although her body had adapted well with collateral circulation. Having done her homework Bertha queried, "Is this not a good thing?" The physician patted her hand and said, "Yes, but you need an immediate quadruple bypass to save your life." Bertha again stated that she was 93 and it was quite acceptable to her to die if that was God's plan. The doctor looked at her and left the room without further discussion. She lay alone for what seemed like a very long time. Finally a nurse came in and said she was being admitted. Bertha shook her head as the nurse said, "It will be fine, you are just scared."

Two days later while on the operating table Bertha experienced a massive heart attack and was repeatedly defibrillated, which left her barely hanging onto life and going in and out of consciousness. Her last words to her daughters before surgery were, "I'm 93 and I have led a good life and it's okay if it is my time to die."

REFLECTIONS ON ISSUES OF CONCERN

1. At what point are people's wishes about their bodies respected?
2. Can a patient advocate really advocate for a patient in a situation like this? Who speaks for the patient who is soft spoken?
3. What is the nurse's responsibility with a patient who has been given an unexpected or terminal diagnosis?
4. Who decides what is best for a patient who is conscious and able to make decisions for himself or herself?
5. How does one's spirituality affect one's views on death and dying? What if this conflicts with the views of the health care staff?

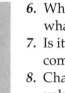

6. What does it take for the health care professional to hear what a patient is saying and honor his or her feelings?
7. Is it necessary to do everything possible when the patient is comfortable with dying?
8. Changing the consciousness around death and dying involves the dying person, the family, and the health care providers. How can you assist in this change?

THE NATURE OF SPIRITUAL PERSPECTIVES

Looking at the nature of spiritual perspectives gives one a broad interpretation of the many and differing characteristics. It gives us a rich tapestry that invites further discovery of the nuances and subtleties of spirituality that far supersede any definition. Looking within itself keeps the mind open to discern insights and grow in understanding. Definitions, especially of spirituality, are incapable of capturing this rich and most incredibly beautiful part of our humanness. Research in its exactness appears unable to capture this rich quality of spiritual perspectives.

With the increasing understanding of the limitations of modern medicine, there has been an increase in research regarding death and the end of life. Whereas modern medicine had put its focus almost exclusively on biomedical management and curing, contemporary medicine is now gradually recognizing the psychospiritual needs of the dying person. In this moment both medical education and medical practice have realized the need to incorporate the understanding of how the dying person can live a richer life not just physically but at all levels of being—physical, psychological, social, and now spiritual (Shimazono, 2009).

Spiritual values often sway the decision-making process of both those dying and their families even though these spiritual values appear to be immaterial when continuation of life-supporting treatment is judged futile. Viewed from a larger perspective these clinical assessments are an invitation to begin to look deeper into spiritual beliefs and values (Ankeny, Clifford, Jordens, Kerridge, & Benson, 2005).

A broad spectrum of spirituality appears at the end of life surrounding the areas of spiritual despair, spiritual work, and spiritual well-being. These areas are further broken down in Table 10.1, "End-of-Life Spectrum of Spirituality." At the end of life the deep-seated significance of spirituality has been established. When a dying person is able to do the necessary spiritual work, the shifts in continuing spiritual health within this spectrum are achievable. Spiritual work is a necessary and vital part of the end of life that is neglected in most frameworks. Improving the interventions aimed at the quality of life and spiritual health is fertile ground for development at the end of life (Williamson, 2006).

Research at Children's Hospital in Boston, Massachusetts, identified the nature and role of spirituality from the parents' perspective at end of life in the pediatric intensive care unit (Robinson Thiel, Backus & Meyer, 2006). The results demonstrated that four explicit spiritual themes come into view: "prayer, faith, access to and care from clergy, and belief in the transcendent quality of the parent–child relationship that endures beyond death" (Robinson Thiel, Backus & Meyer, 2006). Several implicit spiritual themes also emerged, including "insight and wisdom, reliance on values; and virtues such as hope, trust, and love" (Robinson Thiel, Backus & Meyer, 2006). Many parents' spirituality was a source of guidance, reliance, and strength when they had to make end-of-life decisions. Many of the parents experienced the death of their child as a spiritual journey (Robinson Thiel, Backus & Meyer, 2006).

Enhancing the spiritual aspect of dying is quite possibly the most challenging as well as one of the most pertinent aspects of care that is long overdue. Many vital questions remain with respect to end-of-life care and spiritual issues. Efforts have been made to elaborate and deepen the understanding of spiritual well-being using concepts such as dignity, hope, and meaning. Attempts have been made to correlate these constructs with outcomes and variables like acceptance, coping with loss, quality of life during the end of life, and certainly pain control. These are all necessary and vital to our understanding

TABLE 10.1   End-of-Life Spectrum of Spirituality

End-of-Life Spectrum	Characteristics
Spiritual despair	Alienation
	Loss of self
	Dissonance
Spiritual work	Forgiveness
	Self-exploration
	Search for balance
Spiritual well-being	Connection
	Self-actualization
	Consonance

and our ability to give appropriate care. In addition, these issues need to be viewed from faith-based, spirituality-based, and secular perspectives. Expanding the horizon of end-of-life care by addressing the spiritual dimensions has the potential to enhance the quality of life remaining for the dying person while decreasing suffering (Chochinov & Cann, 2005).

Spiritual perspectives from different levels of health care providers extend our understanding about where they are and how they can address this in their practice. Certainly, managed care leaders desire the continuing enhancement of total well-being within a capitated system of care. As a result they must direct their attention to the broad new societal interest surrounding spiritual perspectives and end-of-life care. They need to discover ways to enhance the structure of care through integrating spirituality. Managed care leaders who value their own spirituality and realize the value of spirituality in healing will probably take the lead in this integration. In order to promote individual total well-being, it is fundamental to acknowledge everyone's spiritual dimension. This perspective must acknowledge the spiritual dimension not only in wellness but also in times of crisis, including the fear of death. In the case of health challenges resulting in high health care costs — for example, fear of death, alcoholism, and violence—attention to the spiritual perspectives can assist in decreasing the costs (Hillman, 1997).

Health care providers' perspectives on spirituality are often focused on spiritual care, as seen in the Touhy (2005) study in Boca Raton, Florida. Five major themes emerged from this qualitative study of nursing home health care providers: "honoring the person's dignity, intimate knowing in the nursing home environment, wishing we could do more, personal knowing of self as care giver, and struggling with end of life treatment decisions," with spiritual caring described as "deep personal relationships, holistic care, and support for residents" (Touhy, 2005, p. 27).

Supporting families with end-of-life decisions and having adequate time and staff to give the family and dying person the care they "wished" the staff had time for are important concerns that can be addressed with the *Golden Room*. The staff would be specifically trained and dedicated to have knowledge and compassion and to spend time and be with the person and the family to work through and journey together to the end of life.

Not to be overlooked are the spiritual perspectives of both racial/ ethnic minorities and nonminorities. This spiritual perspective can be revealed in the question, "What determines a good death?" Certainly the answer varies from individual to individual. Yale University conducted focus groups to discover the answer. Within the 10 domains,

Words of Wisdom

"The search for transcendent goals, supported by death awareness, makes life more meaningful. Humans are a meaning-seeking species. When this experience is limited or entirely excluded, one is deprived of one's human heritage."

From Firestone and Catlett (2009, p. xi).

differences were identified in 3 domains: spiritual concerns, cultural concerns, and individuation. The researchers condlued that greater cultural sensitivity and more humane treatment were needed at the end of life for everyone (Tong et al., 2005). Surely a good death is something that everyone is entitled to, regardless of color, creed, race, culture, religious beliefs, and the situation or circumstances.

The elusive nature of spiritual perspectives reflects the grandeur of the universe, the enormity of the realm of spirit, and the difficulty of putting the unknown into the world of form and words. To be in this moment in time with someone is possibly the highest calling of a health care professional. And possibly that is enough. Through the simple action of being with and caring for, we are meeting and even transcending the physical and meeting the dying person and his or her family on the common ground of spiritual awareness (Exhibit 10.1).

SPIRITUAL PERSPECTIVES FROM VARIOUS RELIGIOUS GROUPS

When people are confronted with their mortality, spiritual and religious concerns become the central focus for the vast majority. Everyone is spiritual; this is a universal human attribute. Religion, however, is the more formal structure that expresses a specific doctrine and series of beliefs. Not all people clearly define their belief system or are part of a religious assembly. Many spiritual people do not profess a religion while intense religiosity—ritualistic, habitualistic, formalized behavior—may not appear to express spirituality to others (Olson, 2001).

Religious meanings provide a context for understanding not only death but also life after death (Papadatou, 2009). The three largest monotheistic religions in the United States are Christianity, Islam, and Judaism (Woll, Hinshaw, & Pawlik, 2008). An overview of each in rela-

EXHIBIT 10.1   Research Perspective

Although spiritual care is a core element of palliative care, it remains unclear how this care is perceived and delivered at the end of life. One study explored how clinicians and other health care workers understand and view spiritual care provided to dying patients and their family members. This study was based on qualitative research using key informant interviews and editing analysis with 12 clinicians and other health care workers nominated as spiritual caregivers by dying patients and their family members. Results indicated that being present was a predominant theme, marked by physical proximity and intentionality, or the deliberate ideation and purposeful action of providing care that went beyond medical treatment. Opening eyes was the process by which caregivers became aware of their patient's life course and the individualized experience of their patient's current illness. Participants also described another course of action, which the researchers termed *cocreating*, that was a mutual and fluid activity among patients, family members, and caregivers. Cocreating began with an affirmation of the patient's life experience and led to the generation of a wholistic care plan that focused on maintaining the patient's humanity and dignity. Time was both a facilitator and inhibitor of effective spiritual care. The conclusion of this study was that clinicians and other health care workers consider spiritual care at the end of life as a series of highly fluid interpersonal processes in the context of mutually recognized human values and experiences, rather than a set of prescribed and proscribed roles.

From Daaleman, Usher, Williams, Rawlings, and Hanson (2008).

tion to its spiritual perspectives is presented, followed by a selection of other religions of note.

Christianity

Since the dawn of time each human's existence has ended with death. During the Middle Ages death was consider a natural part of life, certainly universal, and was usually a daily happening. Death was an essential part of life since people believed in an afterlife and an immortal soul. The fate of the person's soul after death depended on how the physical life ended. For instance, in the Old Polish period "good dying" included prayer, penance, alms, and some sort of reconciliation with the physical world. Often, in the Catholic denomination, testaments were drafted consisting of requests for prepaid intercessory prayers and money set aside for the needy. Both Catholics and Protestants had the custom of lavish funerals and the quiet, small funeral requested in some wills was not usually granted by the heirs (Paciorek, 2007).

The Christian religion brings a particular understanding of the ideas of life as God's gift, the individual's responsibility for stewardship of his or her life, each person's wholeness, and the dying process as the doorway to the spiritual life beyond physical life (Stempsey, 1997). Most essential to Christian beliefs and understandings of death and dying are a recognition of God's dominion over the human life, an accepting of suffering associated with Jesus the Christ who is the foundation of Christian hope, and the realization that God's creative and redemptive intention is life (Lustig, 1995).

Christianity has many religious interpretations. For example, Catholics believe that Jesus' grief, suffering, and death were part of God's divine providence. Christ died and rose from the dead. Having this faith allows Catholics to view death as an entry into life with God, who died for them and their sins. Last rites, which includes the sacrament anointing of the sick, provides bodily and spiritual renewal and prepares one for death (Sherman, 2010). It is important that the caregiver summon a priest to perform this end-of-life ritual for practicing Catholics.

Islam (Muslim)

Islam means "submission," while *Muslim* means "one who submits." A Muslim is someone who submits to Allah, the Arabic name for God. Muslims believe in divine predestination and perceive suffering as atonement for their sins. Generally Muslims are uncomfortable with discussing death and inclined to say, "It's in the hands of God." Death is viewed as the beginning of a new, different form of life. Cremation is not acceptable, and burial should occur as soon as possible after death (Sherman, 2010).

Judaism

The Jewish faith believes in affirming life and offering consolation in death. Death is considered inevitable and natural, as it comes from God and therefore should not be feared. People of this faith believe that the soul exists before the body comes into being and continues on after the body dies. Death rituals are designed to help the bereaved to accept the fact that their loved one is gone and to move on. The Jewish funeral is a rite of separation where the rabbi recites prayers expressive of the spirit of the person and the occasion. There is a period of 7 days of mourning. Either burial or cremation is allowed (Sherman, 2010).

Other Religious Perspectives

Native American Spirituality

Native American tribes, such as the Muscogee Creek Tribe in Oklahoma express their spirituality in unique ways. They are open to unexplainable supernatural events and the awareness of spiritual beings—both the good ones and the bad ones. Their religious beliefs hold that spirits exist alongside people. These spirits can both send and receive information to guide and help those on the physical plane. Ongoing though not necessarily constant relationships are the norm with the dead, both with loved ones and others. Being in tune with the spiritual can occur any time in the life cycle. It is particularly apparent in its expression in children and animals (Walker & Thompson, 2009). As with the indigenous Aboriginal people of Australia, models of care and support need to be more culturally friendly and take into consideration both indigenous and Western beliefs. There is a definite need for cultural security, removing system barriers and explaining technoscientific quality, to guarantee that indigenous people can utilize the benefits of modern treatments (Shahid, Bessarab, & Thompson, 2009).

Jehovah's Witnesses

The most common situation relating to death and dying is the Jehovah's Witnesses' refusal of blood when a transfusion is needed. Instead, they ask the health care personnel to offer all the other scientific and medical alternatives. Often the alternatives are not as effective and may fail, causing disability and even death (Smith, 1997). Their deep belief in the body's ability to heal itself and to not accept any foreign substances is a value that the health care personnel need to be aware of to carry out responsible actions and decisions.

Eastern Religions

As the U.S. older adult population increases in cultural diversity, differing perspectives concerning the end of life will become more evident.

Hinduism is a faith that is growing in the United States (Deshpande, Reid, & Roa, 2005). This religion believes in reincarnation, cycles of being born and dying in an infinite series of lives. Karma, every act or thought, has an effect on who that person becomes. Another Eastern religion, Buddhism, does not believe in God or a soul. Buddhists believe in karma and rebirth, like the Hindus. They train their minds to become peaceful and engage that skill as death approaches. At death there is a transfer of consciousness out of the body. Other Eastern religions, such as Confucianism or Taoism, are less prevalent in North America (Sherman, 2010).

European Countries

One's cultural heritage often reflects spiritual perspectives that supersede religion. Hungarian perspectives on end-of-life care, for example, appear to mirror the findings from other European countries concerning death and dying. In Hungary death and dying are taboo topics to talk about. A questionnaire was sent to 29 adult primary care offices with a total of 845 unselected patients. Only 19% said they would prefer to die in a hospital. Care of the dying person, satisfactory relief of symptoms, and the spiritual and psychosocial support of the dying person and his or her family were perceived as not being well attended to in Hungary. Patients' greatest fear was the loss of autonomy and becoming dependent of caregivers (55%) with the second most common fear being pain and suffering (38%; Calkos, Albanese, Buss, Nagy, & Radwany, 2008).

SPIRITUAL HEALTH CARE

It is quite easy, and often is the case, that health care professionals reduce spiritual care to asking, "What is your religion?" or do a spiritual assessment and feel that this is sufficient. This cursory approach is insufficient. Unlike physical and mental care, spiritual care necessitates that the health care providers are comfortable with their own spirituality in order to be of assistance to the dying person and his or her family. We must first begin with ourselves and address our spirituality; in other words, begin near to go far. This is even more interesting because it is uncharted water as far as research goes. Spirituality is an inside job that cannot be measured; only its results can be measured. As health care professionals there are several areas for us to consider as we ourselves move deeper into our spirituality and become comfortable: vibrational essence, open heart, authentic language, and intuitive knowing.

Vibrational Essence

When we rise above our religious dogmas and practices we discover spiritual commonalities. It is here that we can meet, where the river meets the sea, in oneness of body, oneness of mind, and oneness of spirit. Here in our vibrational essence we discover an open heart, authentic language, and intuitive knowing. From this vantage point we come together to create a place for death with dignity: the *Golden Room*.

Reawakening our consciousness of vibrational essence has long been seen as a time-bound process that, depending on the teaching, can take weeks, months, or even years. No matter what our minds or the minds of others say, we can begin now, for in reality it is here that we live, breathe, and have our being. It is here, now, in this moment. It is as simple as that. This is our moment, a one-of-a-kind moment that is and will be like no other. So is the next moment and the next moment and the next moment. Each moment is fresh, new, never to be repeated again. Although all moments may appear to be the same, they are not. In often subtle ways each moment is different. Our mind simply puts moments together in groups for ease of storing and categorizing. As a result we think they are all the same. They are not. This being the case, each moment is truly a rare and precious gift in its uniqueness. As we begin to realize this phenomenon, our attitude toward the present moment begins to change regardless of what we are doing. We begin to see and feel each moment, savor each moment as a special God-created opportunity to express and experience oneness with God and all creation. We begin to realize the sacredness of life. Within this realization of the sacredness of life the concept of a place for death with dignity, the *Golden Room*, was born.

Being here in this moment is as simple as turning your attention. You are reading. Look up and look at something in your surroundings. Look at it as if you have never seen it before. Look at the detail, no thinking, simply looking. Take your time and actually do this now. Did you do it? This is more powerful if you experience it rather than intellectualize it. You turned your attention away from the book onto something else. Being in the moment is that simple. It is turning your attention away from the meandering thoughts of the mind onto something else. So often we get caught in the treadmill of the mind's machinations and we fail to see what is around us. We get lost in the mind and miss the incredible world unfolding in this moment. This is where we live—in this moment. When we spend so much time in our minds, we miss the incredible experience of physical life. *The Golden Room* is a place where health care professionals assist the patient and his or her family to spend more and more of their time in the present moment.

This moment is the place of discovery, life, moving into solutions, comfort, dignity, and respect. From this vantage point we begin to live and experience life on its terms as we move though the dying experience. We discover that physical death is not to be feared and pushed under the table. Death is a normal part of the physical life experience. In this moment we discover that time appears to stand still in a good way. Everything that needs to be accomplished is accomplished; everything that needs to be said is said, as it is all spirit led.

Living in the moment is the spirit-led life that the masters, mystics, and great teachers have talked about for centuries. Being in the moment is actually showing up in your life, experiencing the moment and acknowledging your feelings to yourself. This is an internal process because they are your feelings and no one else can feel them for you. Your feelings are based on your prior experiences, which are often so far removed and different from the current situation that you are not conscious of them anymore. The present situation brings up that feeling memory. We are reacting to a past feeling rather than the present situation. To respond to the present situation we need to turn our attention to this moment, breathe easily, and allow ourselves to take in without judgment exactly what is happening. It is as if we are stepping behind our minds into the universal mind of God . . . the larger perspective. Not only the clients or patients but also the health care professionals who work in the *Golden Room* have experienced and are increasingly living in this present moment. With gentle guidance they can meet the dying loved one and family where they are and help them return to this essence of being.

Open Heart

As we as health care providers begin to live more and more in the present moment and are sensitive to our feelings and where they are located in our bodies, we begin to discover the feelings of our heart. We are aware when our hearts are heavy or light, when they open up or shut down. Not only do we become sensitive to our heart and feelings when we focus on them, but also we begin to feel our heart responding at different times during the day spontaneously in the background. Our vibrational essence is speaking to us through the shift in the feelings of our heart . . . felt oneness with being. As we observe this happening there is a realization that this presence, this vibrational essence we know of as God, is speaking to us and guiding us. We simply need to feel, acknowledge, and take action to move forward. *The Golden Room* is a place for an opportunity to take this closer walk with God as we move through the experience of death and dying.

Authentic Language

As our heart opens another aspect of being in the present moment emerges. We begin to speak with clarity and deep wisdom from an inner place of authentic language. The words begin to come through our minds rather than from our minds. The words are appropriate and reflect the larger perspective of what is occurring. The words are acknowledging and comforting and seem to greet and stir the vibrational essence of those who hear them. This sounds like magic, but it is not. It is simply a gift of being in the present moment. We all have experienced times when the words seemed to flow from deep inside. We can tap this source through being in the present moment.

Intuitive Knowing

Quite possibly the most awesome power of present-moment living is the awakening of our intuitive knowing. We call this our sixth sense. It is that and more. This is the knowledge of the universal mind of God flowing through us to guide and assist us in our actions. This knowing is beyond our physical mind and taps into the entire resources of the universe. Time collapses into the present moment, and everything that is needed is revealed. Our intuition is so far beyond our mind that it is impossible to explain yet incredible to experience. Suffice it to say, "It is a God thing." When we are in the present moment we allow ourselves to do what we feel we need to be doing and to say what we are led to say. And we are not concerned with the outcome. The outcome takes care of itself. We focus on being, moving, and acting in the present moment. We often see this take place in situations where things are happening so fast that there is no time to think; instead, we just do. There is no mind here, simply doing as if the body had a mind of its own. Afterwards the mind jumps in to explain what happened. How many times have we had the sense of knowing that we needed to say or do something but hesitated from fear of the outcome or someone's reaction? These inner promptings are our intuitive knowing trying to come through. This knowingness becomes stronger only when we acknowledge it and follow it. There are no wrong decisions here, no second guessing. When we live in the present moment, things just are and we respond to what is presented to us.

In a place for death with dignity, the *Golden Room*, our intuitive knowing comes through in many ways. We might feel the need to gently rub someone's arm or massage the calves of his or her legs. We might offer a drink or encourage him or her to roll over. We might suggest that the family get some rest on the extra bed that is in the room especially for them. We might turn on some soft music that the patient enjoys, or we might simply say, "It's okay now, you can rest, I will be here watching and waiting." We might offer some pain medication.

THE DEATH EXPERIENCE FROM A SPIRITUAL PERSPECTIVE

Everything in the physical and mental worlds has its limitations. Living in the present moment, we experience minideaths all the time. With each breath we breathe in and breathe out, we turn to the next breath without holding on to the last breath. We literally die to each breath as we turn to the next. Our physical life is a series of minideaths: as we leave childhood, graduate from school, leave home, marry, divorce, move, change jobs, lose our gloves, lose the movement in our fingers, or lose our balance. As we embrace life in the moment it is with the deepening realization that nothing lasts forever. Life is here for us to experience in this moment. Life is neither good nor bad; it is simply an experience. When we move beyond the good–bad dichotomy we discover a joy and spontaneity for living, almost an excitement to discover what will happen next.

When we are born, our first physical act is to take a breath in, to inhale. When we die our last physical act is to let the breath out, to exhale. Dying is a simple physical process of exhaling. We practice for the death experience hundreds of times during each day. When we release all the mind games and fears and simply are in the present moment, death becomes not an enemy to fight but rather a friend to embrace.

SUMMARY

Spirituality appears to be larger and more encompassing than religious rituals, customs, and mores. From this larger awareness, commonalities between religions begin to become apparent. It is from this place of common ground based on basic values, including human dignity, the sacredness of all life, care, nonviolence, selflessness, and compassion, that we can begin to negotiate the method and comportment to provide care. This supersedes the still-existing conflicts and differences (Ankeny et al., 2005). In essence we are taking the natural spiritual concepts of death and dying and reinvesting them in the dying process as being available to the vast majority rather than the minority of people. This is the place where the *Golden Room* begins and has its being.

REFERENCES

Ankeny, R., Clifford, R., Jordens, C., Kerridge, I., & Benson, R. (2005, December). Religious perspectives on withdrawal of treatment from patients with multiple organ failure. *Medical Journal of Australia*, 183(11–12), 616–621.

Calkos, A., Albanese, T., Buss, C., Nagy, L., & Radwany, S. (2008). Hungarians' perspectives on end-of-life care. *Journal of Palliative Medicine, 11*(8), 1083–1087.

Chochinov, H., & Cann, B. (2005). Interventions to enhance the spiritual aspects of dying. *Journal of Palliative Medicine, 8*(Suppl. 1), S103–S105.

Daaleman T. P., Usher, B. M., Williams, S. W., Rawlings, J., & Hanson, L. C. (2008). An exploratory study of spiritual care at the end of life. *Annals of Family Medicine, 6*(5), 406–411.

Deshpande, O., Reid, M., & Roa, A. (2005). Attitudes of Asian Indian Hindus toward end-of-life care. *Journal of the American Geriatrics Society, 53*(1), 131–135.

Firestone, R. W., & Catlett, J. (2009). *Beyond death anxiety*. New York: Springer Publishing Company.

Hillman, G. (1997). The place of spirituality in managed care: Attending to spiritual needs can help managed care systems achieve their goals. *Health Progress, 78*(1), 43–46.

Lustig, B. (1995). Suffering, sovereignty, and the purposes of God: Christian convictions and medical killing. *Christian Bioethics, 1*(3), 249–255.

Olson, M. (2001). *Healing the dying* (2nd ed.). Albany, NY: Delmar Press.

Paciorek, M. (2007). The relation to the soul and body in the "good death" category in the light of Old Polish manuals, guides and wills. *Med Nowozytna, 14*(1–2), 43–54. Retrieved March 1, 2010, from http://www.ncbi,nlm.nih.gov/pubmed?term="Paciorek

Papadatou, D. (2009). *In the face of death*. New York: Springer Publishing Company.

Robinson, M., Thiel, M., Backus, M., & Meyer, E. (2006). Matters of spirituality at end of life in the pediatric intensive care unit. *Pediatrics, 118*(3), e719–e729.

Shahid, S., Bessarab, D., & Thompson, S. (2009). Understanding, beliefs and perspectives of Aboriginal people in Western Australia about cancer and its impact on access to cancer services. *BMC Health Services Research, 31*(9), 132.

Sherman, D. W. (2010). "Culture & Spirituality as Domains of Quality Palliative Care" In M. Matzo & D. Sherman (Eds.), *Palliative care nursing* (3rd ed.). New York: Springer Publishing Company.

Shimazono, S. (2009). Cancer treatment and death studies. *Gan To Kagaku Ryoho, 36*(10), 1597–1601.

Smith, M. (1997). Ethical perspectives on Jehovah's Witnesses' refusal of blood. *Cleveland Clinic Journal of Medicine, 64*(9), 475–481.

Stempsey, W. (1997). End-of-life decisions: Christian perspectives. *Christian Bioethics, 3*(3), 249–261.

Tong, E., McCraw, S., Dobihal, E., Baggish, R., Cherlin, E., & Bradley, E. (2005). What is a good death? Minority and non-minority perspectives. *Journal of Palliative Care, 19*(3), 168–175.

Touhy, C. (2005). Spiritual care: End of life in a nursing home. *Journal of Gerontological Nursing, 31*(9), 27–35.

Walker, A., & Thompson, T. (2009). Muscogee Creek spirituality and meaning of death. *Omega (Westport), 59*(2), 129–146.

Williamson, A. L. (2006). Perspectives on spirituality at the end of life: A meta-summary. 4(4), 207–217.

Woll, M., Hinshaw, D., & Pawlik, T. (2008). Spirituality and religion in the care of surgical oncology patients with life-threatening or advanced illnesses. *Annals of Oncology, 15*(11), 3048–3057.

11 Palliative Care to Hospice to the Golden Room

If you want others to be happy . . . practice compassion. If you want to be happy . . . practice compassion.

—His Holiness the Dalai Lama

*H*AROLD'S STORY   *Harold is a 62-year-old chronic smoker with bladder cancer. He has been in and out of treatment for 2 years and was recently readmitted for a renal calculus and now has obstructed urine flow. Six months ago Harold underwent a bladder resection; now the cancer has metastasized to other organs. If he were healthy and viable he would have another surgery to remove the kidney stone; however, he is not strong enough to survive surgery. His urologist has come to an impasse at treatment and asked the invasive radiologist to insert a urethral stent to facilitate urine flow. Since it is a weekend, the radiologist feels the need to bring in a team of three people to assist with stint insertion. The following Tuesday, the patient is worse, urine flow has diminished, and the stint has dislodged. Magnetic resonance imaging (MRI) is planned to assess the further deterioration and to determine the location of the obstructing kidney stone.*

REFLECTIONS ON ISSUES OF CONCERN

1. Are there legal implications of not proceeding to do more invasive care on this patient?
2. When can the medical team decide that this patient has reached the stage of futility?
3. Can and should this medical team recommend transfer out of acute care into another option: palliative care, hospice, or the *Golden Room*?
4. Are there certain criteria that signify the time for transfer to palliative care?

End-of-life issues have made tremendous strides during the past 45 years. The history of modern end-of-life care is rich with activity, as shown in the chronology in Table 11.1. The amazing fact is that so much has happened within a short time frame.

Here we are, 43 years after the inception of the concept of hospice in the United States, and we are still working on offering death with dignity. Yes, we have made progress. Now we are ready for the next two steps: (1) shifting the consciousness and comfortableness around the end of life, and (2) making *Golden Rooms* available across the United States.

TABLE 11.1   Chronology of the History of End-of-Life Care in the Modern Era

Year	Event
1967	Dame Cicely Saunders established the first modern hospice: St. Christopher's, London, England. She launched the hospice concept in the United States on a lecture tour.
1969	Dr. Elisabeth Kübler-Ross published the first comprehensive end-of-life book, *On Death and Dying*, beginning the U.S. grassroots movement.
1978	National Hospice Organization (NHO) is established. The first hospice in the United States is established in New Haven, Connecticut.
1980	A 2-year demonstration project of 27 hospices is passed by Congress to study improved health care for terminally ill patients.
1982	Medicare Part A: Medicare Hospice Benefit is passed by Congress.
1987	Hospice Nurses Association (HNA) begins.
1990	International standards defining hospice and palliative care are set by the World Health Organization (WHO).
1994	First hospice specialist nurses are certified by the National Board for Certification of Hospice Nurses.
1997	The HNA becomes the Hospice and Palliative Nurses Association.
1999	Hospice and Palliative Nurses certification is established.
2000	National Hospice and Palliative Care Organization morphs out of the NHO.
2010	Death with dignity: *The Golden Room* is proposed

From History of end-of-life care, End of Life: A nurse's guide to compassionate care (2007). Lippincott Williams & Wilkins. Ambler, PA, p. 3

PALLIATIVE CARE

Palliative care is the medical subspecialty focused on relief of the pain, symptoms, and stress of serious illness. The goal is to ensure the highest quality of life possible for patients and their families. Palliative medicine treats serious illness regardless of the prognosis, and patients can receive it at any point in their illness, with or without curative treatment.

It is expected that by 2030 the number of older Americans will have more than doubled to 70 million—or one in every five Americans. With the availability of advanced medical technologies older adults are expected to live longer but often with serious, chronic, and costly illnesses. Since it improves physical and psychological symptoms, caregiver well-being, and patient, family, and doctor communication, palliative medicine is widely viewed as an important solution to the mounting problems faced by patients, families, and the health care system (Goldsmith, Dietrich, Qinging Du, & Morrison, 2008).

Palliative Care Defined

The World Health Organization (2002) provides this definition of palliative care:

> *Palliative Care is an approach that improves the quality of life of patients and their families facing the problem associated with life-threatening illness, through the prevention and relief of suffering by means of early identification and impeccable assessment and treatment of pain and other problems, physical, psychosocial and spiritual.*

A similar definition is given by the American Geriatrics Society. They define palliative care as care directed toward the quality of life of patients who are dying, including the relief of pain and other symptoms; attention to the psychological, emotional, social, and spiritual needs of the patient; and the provision of support for the dying patient and the patient's family (American Geriatrics Society, 2007).

Palliative care

- Provides relief from pain and other distressing symptoms
- Affirms life and regards dying as a normal process
- Intends to neither hasten nor postpone death

- Integrates the psychological and spiritual aspects of patient care
- Offers a support system to help patients live as actively as possible until death
- Offers a support system to help the family cope during the patient's illness and in their own bereavement
- Uses a team approach to address the needs of patients and their families, including bereavement counseling, if indicated
- Enhances quality of life and may also positively influence the course of illness
- Is applicable early in the course of illness, in conjunction with other therapies that are intended to prolong life, such as chemotherapy or radiation therapy, and includes those investigations needed to better understand and manage distressing clinical complications.

Regional Differences

It is amazing how geography matters in the location and numbers of palliative care facilities. In the South, for example, one is much less likely to find a hospital with a palliative care program. In regions where there are only small hospitals (fewer than 50 beds), chances of having access to palliative care are extremely low:

- The lowest prevalence of hospital palliative care programs is found in Mississippi (10%), Alabama (16%), Oklahoma (19%), Nevada (23%), and Wyoming (25%).
- The highest prevalence of hospital palliative care programs is found in Vermont (100%), Montana (88%), New Hampshire (85%), the District of Columbia (80%), and South Dakota (78%; "America's care of serious illness).

The Rationale for Palliative Care

There are currently 36 million Americans over age 65; of these, 90% have one chronic illness, and more than 77% have two or more chronic conditions (Robert Wood Johnson Foundation, 1996). Despite the goals for increasing accessibility of end-of-life care, oftentimes these end of life care facilities go unused. Exhibit 11.1 details some reasons why this occurs.

As the study discussed in Exhibit 11.1 shows, of the three top reasons for hospice to not be used, two are physician-based: reluctance to make a referral and lack of information about availability and suitability. The

EXHIBIT 11.1   Research Perspective

Supporters of Life-Affirming Care at End of Life (SOLACE) is a coalition of interdisciplinary professionals dedicated to improving end-of-life care. The objectives of a SOLACE survey were to identify and describe (1) professionals' perceptions about barriers related to hospice and palliative care, (2) professionals' opinions about barriers related to dying at home, (3) professionals' perceptions about barriers related to advance directives, and (4) relationships between professionals and their perceived barriers to advance directives and hospice and palliative care. A survey questionnaire solicited responses from professionals on palliative care, dying at home, and advance directives. Measures that assessed obstacles to palliative care were modified from previous studies to yield composite barrier scores. From a sample of a variety of participants at a national conference on palliative care ($n = 200$), 101 subjects returned questionnaires (51%), yielding 100 usable completed forms from attendees who demonstrated an interest in palliative care and, in some cases, a high level of personal or professional experience. Survey results were analyzed to observe respondents' perceptions concerning barriers related to advance directives and the delivery of palliative care. Of the 13 obstacle statements, results show that respondents rated the top three barriers to palliative care as (1) physician reluctance to make referrals, (2) physician lack of familiarity with availability and suitability of hospice, and (3) association of hospice with death.

From Feeg and Elebiary (2005).

third reason could be either physician-, family-, or patient-based: concern about the association of death with hospice. All these reasons speak to the need for better education and the underlying need for shifting the consciousness around the end of life.

Goals of Palliative Care

For patients with active, progressive, far-advanced disease, the goals of palliative care are, according to the International Association of Hospice and Palliative Care ([IAHPC], 2008),

- To provide relief from pain and other physical symptoms
- To maximize the quality of life
- To provide psychosocial and spiritual care
- To provide support to help the family during the patient's illness and bereavement

As is evident from the preceding information, palliative care provides high-quality care during the final phase of the dying process, be it days or hours. Any yet it can also be incorporated into care before all medical alternatives have been exhausted. Historically, palliative care began with the belief that the terminally ill were not receiving optimal care. Today, modern palliative care provides active and holistic care that complements the active treatment of traditional medicine. This holistic care includes better pain and symptom control as well as a deeper appreciation of the psychosocial aspects of care. Palliative care calls for highly trained doctors, nurses, and interprofessional support-

EXHIBIT 11.2   Research Perspective

Australian researchers described the qualitatively different ways nurses understood their experience of being a palliative care nurse. A phenomenographical study of 15 Australian nurses caring for people in a specialist palliative care unit identified and described five ways of understanding the experience of being a palliative care nurse:

- Doing everything you can
- Developing closeness
- Working as a team
- Creating meaning about life
- Maintaining oneself

Conclusion: The palliative care nurses involved in this research understood their experience as journeying with their patients through the final phases of the person's life. The journey involved the patient, his or her family, and members of the health care team. The journey was described further as a process of personal development that influenced how the nurses constructed meaning about life and maintained a sense of self.

From Barnard, Hollingum, and Hartfiel (2006).

ing health care teams (IAHPC, 2008; see (Exhibit 11.2). In the research discussed in Exhibit 11.2 the palliative care nurses integrated their experience as journeying with their patients in the last phases of their physical life.

MEDICATING FOR SYMPTOMS

There is a continuum between the goals of comfort and function in palliative care that begins with comfort and function as equal priorities and sedation considered as unacceptable. As disease progresses, the patient's goals and preferences turn to coping with the loss of function caused by the disease and acceptance of symptom relief interventions or unintentional sedation from the disease or its therapies. As patients approach the end of life, they may need intentional sedation for the relief of refractory symptoms. Palliative care clinicians should become comfortable with the ethical justification and technical expertise needed to provide this essential, extraordinary care to the small but deserving number of patients in whom routine and infrequent sedation does not adequately relieve their suffering (Levy & Cohen, 2005). Table 11.2 details categories of intentional sedation for the relief of refractory symptoms.

Becoming comfortable with intentional sedation at the end of life takes more than a cursory thought and decision. It needs to be carefully reflected on and questioned until the palliative nurse can be part of the solution and not continue the problem because of because of beliefs and attitudes. This is an example of a type of question that can be more easily resolved with a shifting of consciousness and the ability to express one's feelings about it.

Medications such as morphine or hydromorphone are also used for pain. Lorazepam (Ativan) or haloperidol may be used for anxiety,

TABLE 11.2   Categories of Intentional Sedation for the Relief of Refractory Symptoms

Routine	Medications used to induce and maintain a level of sedation that relieves the patient's physical and existential symptoms
Infrequent	Patient PCA pump or prn requests
Extraordinary	Use of continuous infusions of midazolam, thiopental, and propofol can relieve refractory symptoms in most patients in their final days of life

agitation, and delirium. The type of drug tends to vary from one agency to another.

MEDICAL CODES AND BILLING

Palliative care services are generally coded and billed by evaluation and management service on the basis of time spent, symptoms managed, and/or the care coordinated. If and when nurses bill for time spent, documentation in the medical record should reflect total time spent as well as the clinical focus of the timed efforts, that is, coordination of care, end-of-life counseling, or evaluation of medication needs and adjustment.

NEED FOR SPECIALISTS

According to the Center to Advance Palliative Care (CAPC), on the basis of an analysis of the latest data released from the 2008 American Hospital Association (AHA) "Annual Survey of Hospitals," U.S. hospitals continue to implement palliative care programs at a rapid pace. A clinical palliative care program existed in more than 31% (1,299) of 4,136 hospitals appropriate for palliative care in 2008. This number reflects an increase from 632 programs in 2000 (CAPC, 2010).

Most significantly, hospitals with over 50 beds—the most likely to have a program—show a penetration of 47%. Palliative care represents a paradigm shift in how we treat serious illness in America. Ten years ago there were almost no hospital palliative care programs in the United States, but now there are many (CAPC, n.d.).

Of the 4,136 hospitals appropriate for palliative care programs,

- 31% have a program
- 47% of those with over 50 beds have a program
- 77% of those with over 250 beds (large hospitals) have a program

Features commonly associated with hospitals that provide a palliative care consultation service are

- Joint Commission on Accreditation of Healthcare Organizations accreditation
- Cancer program approved by the American College of Surgeons
- Council of Teaching Hospitals (COTH) member hospital

- Catholic church operated
- Large size (i.e., over 250 beds)

Additional data indicate that in states where there is greater access to palliative care programs, patients

- Are less likely to die in the hospital
- Experience fewer intensive care unit/critical care unit admissions in the last 6 months of life
- Spend less time in an intensive care unit/critical care unit in the last 6 months of life (CAPC, n.d.)

A fundamental issue affecting the ability to offer end-of-life care is the lack of qualified, certified physicians and nurses in palliative practice. In 2007, there were 2,883 physicians board-certified in palliative medicine (1 physician per 31,000 persons living with serious and life-threatening illness, or 1 physician per 432 Medicare deaths from chronic illness). In comparison, there are 16,800 cardiologists (1 per 71 heart attack victims) and 10,000 oncologists (1 per 145 patients newly diagnosed with cancer). The highest rates of board-certified palliative medicine physicians are in Hawaii, the District of Columbia, Alaska, New Mexico, and Colorado. The lowest rates are in Mississippi, Arkansas, Nebraska, Idaho, and South Dakota (CAPC, n.d.).

HOSPICE TODAY IN THE UNITED STATES

Hospice is quite possibly the best-kept secret for making an exit from physical life that is as gentle as possible; it is only now spreading to some parts of the country. Since its inception in the 1960s, when Dame Cicely Sanders brought the concept from the United Kingdom, U.S. hospice services have grown and flourished in most parts of the country to some degree. Probably everyone has heard the name *hospice* and has a general knowledge that this "care" is available for the dying. Usually people erroneously think that dying "naturally" means feeling pain and hunger and is not really too pleasant, although people are around to talk the family through this. Most people do not know what is available to them nor have they explored this option. Generally it's only when one is faced with their own mortality or that of a close friend or relative that they recognize the need for this new knowledge.

The mission, vision, and actions of hospice as stated by the IAHPC are as follows:

> *Our Mission is to collaborate and work to improve the quality of life of patients with advanced life-threatening conditions and their families, by advancing hospice and palliative care programs, education, research, and favorable policies around the world. (http://www.hospicecare.com/ Organisation/Org.htm#Mission)*

Their vision is "to help to increase and optimize the availability of and access to hospice and palliative care for patients and their families throughout the world" (http://www.hospicecare.com/Organisation/ Org.htm#Mission).

The mission and vision are achieved through the following actions:

- "Facilitating and providing palliative care education and training opportunities for care providers
- Acting as an information resource for professionals, health care providers and policy makers
- Developing collaborative strategies for hospice and palliative care providers, organizations, institutions and individuals."

America is doing a mediocre job of caring for its most seriously ill and vulnerable hospitalized patients. To improve this, palliative care programs are being put into place at a rapid pace in U.S. hospitals.

Hospice and Palliative Care

When one looks at the actual definitions of hospice and palliative care, a fuller picture of what this entails begins to unfold. Hospice and palliative care are active, not passive, care of persons with progressive and incurable disease. The meaning and use of hospice can vary greatly from country to country, from a general philosophy of care, to a specific type of setting, to unpaid volunteers giving the care, to care in the final days of life (IAHPC, 2008).

At present there are thousands of hospice sites in America. These include freestanding agencies, in-home programs, volunteer programs, and those associated with a hospital. Generally, there are two types of hospice. The first type is donation driven and all-volunteer except for paid registered nurses. All personnel receive special and ongoing training. The family does not pay for the registered nurse or any of the caregivers to come into the home. The hospice receives its funding from contributions by family, friends, and grants. The second type is similar except that the funding is primarily from Medicare and private insurance along with some voluntary contributions.

Hospice Standing Orders

In most hospice situations, nurses act from a series of standing orders. The numbers and scope of orders vary from place to place but generally cover the same situations. Table 11.3 details the types and range of hospice standing orders. The range of hospice standing orders is aimed at comfort and supporting the dying patient to have an end of life that is as physically comfortable as possible.

TABLE 11.3   Hospice Standing Orders

Order	Specifics
Certification date	Gives date range from 1 day up to 6 months life expectancy
Medical equipment	Affords nurse choice of mechanical assistance devices such as shower chair, nebulizer, suction, oxygen for short of breath, and so on
Urinary	Foley catheter size range and irrigation protocol
Skin care	Range of medications to use for decubitus ulcers
Bowels	Lists suppositories and medications for constipation or diarrhea
Nausea and ingestion	Medications such as compazine, raglan, omeprazole ordered
Agitation, confusion, or anxiety	What to look for and range of medications to choose from when patient demonstrates these symptoms
Congestion or cough	Medications such as hycodan, Robitussin, albuterol inhaler offered
Sleep	Hypnotics to deal with sleep deprivation
Seizures	Diazepam with specific dose range and time span stated
Elevated temperature	Range of doses of Tylenol or ibuprofen

Words of Wisdom

"In the modern hospice movement and in Palliative Care, helping severely ill and dying patients to have a 'good end of life' and a 'good death' has high priority. The concept of a 'good death' reflects the corresponding ideal of a 'good dying.'"

From Steffen-Bürgi (2009, p. 371).

THE GOLDEN ROOM AND HOSPICE

With hospice and palliative care now becoming an actual part of contemporary end-of-life care and gaining increasing recognition, it is time to familiarize practitioners and the public with additional options. *The Golden Room* may be one solution to move palliative care and hospice to the next level of recognition and familiarity in America. This solution moves into the heart of acceptance of palliative care and hospice since it deals with shifting how people view the end of life and feel about both others' and their own death, something that is often seen as very far away. In truth no one knows the exact time and day of his or her death. Death even when expected at the end of life is still unexpected. There is always a glimmer of hope that somehow this will pass and one will wake up to things as normal, with this being a bad dream. Even when death is imminent few people actually feel the peace that passes understanding and are able to grow through (not go through) the death of a loved one. The number of these people is growing.

Although death with dignity is aimed at the dying person, the family has to deal with their feelings during the dying process. These feelings frequently determine the course of the dying process. To begin a discussion of death and dying within a family, within a community, within a profession is to begin to deal with these illusory feelings of immortality of oneself and others. The dying process and ultimately death is a unique experience that one finally must go through by oneself. The way can be made much more honorable and dignified when not only the dying person but also the family has the love and support of a gentle process that recognizes and supports each person wherever he or she is at in understanding and dealing with the dying process. This recognition and support are inclusive rather than exclusive, inclusive in that it recognizes that this experience and these circumstances are a natural part of the human life cycle, exclusive in that each person and each family will experience it differently so that no book, no lecture, no experience can really prepare anyone—the dying person, the family, or the health care professional—as to what will transpire. To generalize would be to trivialize a person's existence. Each person is unique, and his or her life is significant and important, as is his or her death. Opening this discussion and introspection is a point of monumental growth and acceptance.

This shift in consciousness to speaking about the unspeakable rather than waiting until it is upon us is a tremendous step in openness and dealing with our inner fears so that the things once thought of as demons become angels of love and understanding. It seems most timely to create greater public awareness and promote acceptance of death and dying as a normal part of the physical life cycle. *The Golden Room* offers a place for death with dignity, an alternative currently not available to most people in nursing homes and acute care hospitals.

SUMMARY

Palliative care to hospice to the *Golden Room* represents an ever-expanding spiral of growth in our understanding and appreciation. There is beauty, complexity, dignity, and deep honor in being with those dying and their families at this sacred time when the veil between two worlds becomes very thin as one precious life-form is transformed from the known physical into the unknown dimension. This is a natural progression in our growth in understanding and awareness of the balance and cycle of life. *Golden Rooms* represent our legacy to our children as the next step in our continuing growth in understanding our place in all of creation.

REFERENCES

American Geriatrics Society. (2007). *Position statement on the care of dying patients* [Electronic version]. Retrieved May 18, 2010, from http://www.americangeriatrics.org

Barnard, A., Hollingum, C., & Hartfiel, B. (2006). Going on a journey: Understanding palliative care nursing. *International Journal of Palliative Nursing, 12*(1), 6–12.

Feeg, V. D., & Elebiary, H. (2005). Exploratory study on end-of-life issues: Barriers to palliative care and advance directives. *American Journal of Hospice and Palliative Care, 22*(2), 119–124.

Goldsmith, B., Dietrich, J., Qinging Du, M. S., & Morrison, S. (2008). Variability in access to hospital palliative care in the United States. *Journal of Palliative Medicine, 11*(8), 1094–1102.

Concepts of palliative care, End of Life: A nurse's guide to compassionate care (2007). Lippincott Williams & Wilkins. Ambler, PA., p. 3

International Association of Hospice and Palliative Care. (2008). *IAHPC manual of palliative care* (2nd ed.) [Electronic version]. Retrieved May 5, 2010, from http://www.hospicecare.com/manual/toc-main.html

Levy, M. H., & Cohen, S. D. (2005). Sedation for the relief of refractory symptoms in the imminently dying: A fine intentional line. *Seminars in Oncology, 32*(2), 237–246.

Robert Wood Johnson Foundation. (1996). *Chronic care in America: A 21 century challenge.* Princeton, NJ: Author.

Steffen-Bürgi, B. (2009). Ideas about a "good death." *Palliative Care Nursing, 22*(5), 371–378.

World Health Organization. (2002). *National cancer control programmes: Policies and managerial guidelines* (2nd ed.). Geneva, Switzerland : Author. Retrieved April 21, 2010, from http://www.who.int/cancer/palliative/definition/en/

Retrieved May 3, 2010, from http://www.hospicecare.com/Organisation/Org.htm#Mission

Center to Advance Palliative Care. News Release. http://www.capc.org/news-and-events/releases/news-release-4-14-08

"America's care of serious illness." Retrieved August 16, 2010, from http://www.capc.org/reportcard/findings

Part III

Implementation Steps

*Guide to Implementing the Golden Room
Concept with Health Professionals*

It doesn't matter how slowly you go
As long as you do not stop.
                    —Confucius

*D*r. WILLARD'S STORY   *Dr. Willard was a family physician for
over 50 years. He advocated a low-fat, high-fiber diet, moderate
exercise, and nutritional supplements for a strong base for good
general health. He was ahead of his time, and his patients loved
him. He pretty much walked his talk for most of his life. At age 68
he fell off the wagon. Over the next 10 years he gained 35 pounds,
exercised infrequently and with increasing difficulty, had high blood
pressure, and appeared to be aging rapidly with increasing ached
and pains. He decided to take action and began a rigorous exercise
program and changed his diet. One morning while jogging he
experienced mild chest pains. Being close to home he walked home
slowly and immediately called 911. The paramedics arrived, took
his blood pressure, put on cardiac leads, started an IV, transferred
him to a stretcher, and took him to the hospital.*

*Having lived alone since his wife died 8 years earlier, Dr. Willard
was now at the mercy of the very institution he had worked so hard
to prevent his patients from experiencing. He had no children and
no close relatives. The emergency room (ER), though familiar to him,
was now seen from an entirely different perspective. Although he
knew the drill, now that this was happening to him it was completely
different. He felt scared and alone. The ER staff were professional,
efficient, and friendly but had no time to spend with him. He was
quickly assessed with an electrocardiogram (EKG) and blood gases
and stabilized with medications. A cardiac consult was done, and he
was then sent to a medical floor for observation and to wait for
additional testing the next morning. That night Dr. Willard slept
poorly in spite of a sleeping pill, tossing and turning and aware of
all the leads on his chest and the lights from the EKG machine and
the IV in his arm. More testing in the morning revealed blocked*

cardiac arteries with collateral circulation and the need for an immediate quadruple bypass. Dr. Willard reluctantly agreed and signed the papers, having never expected to have this happen to him.

The next morning during surgery Dr. Willard went into cardiac arrest two times, necessitating cardiac massage and ventilation. Finally arriving in the cardiac intensive care he was put on the critical list; the next 24 hours would determine his prognosis. Many lab tests later he began to stabilize, only to have respiratory distress; he was immediately put on a ventilator. His advance directives were in the chart, but no one was there as an advocate for him. He had assumed that everyone knew him, and he had made his wishes known quite vocally in the hospital. Massive IV antibiotics were started to quell the infection in his lung, and a nasogastric tube was inserted. Dr. Willard shifted in and out of consciousness and was restrained to keep him from pulling on his tubes. His medical care team felt sad that he of all people had come to this. For over a week Dr. Willard's body struggled to overcome the infection. Finally one of the cardiac consultants, upon reading the chart and realizing who this patient was, ordered that the ventilator be discontinued. Within 2 hours after its removal Dr. Willard coded. Being a Do Not Resuscitate patient he was allowed to die; a nurse and a physician were both there, waiting to document the time.

REFLECTIONS ON ISSUES OF CONCERN

1. As a health professional what are your expectations as to how you will die?
2. What have you done to ensure that this happens?
3. What responsibility do you have to your profession to create a space for death with dignity for your patients?
4. How can you best guide others to a dignified death?

Health professionals are in the unique place to be able to create change within the health care system. One imperative, as you have already read, is the escalating necessity for death with dignity for the increasing aging population at the end of life.

PALLIATIVE CARE AND HOSPICE NURSES

Probably the nurses in the most unique position to be able to understand not only the physical dying process but also the consciousness that accompanies it are palliative and hospice nurses. Dealing with end-of-life issues on a daily basis, these nurses have discovered not just through education but even more through experience and self-reflection the extreme importance of this last journey that each person makes and how important it is for the dying and their families that it be completed with dignity and grace.

From this pool of specialty nurses *Golden Rooms* will first draw their staff. And these seasoned nurses will aid the implementation of *Golden Rooms* with suggestions for refinement and needs. How often has one of them said, "If only we had . . . it would make this a much easier and smoother process?"

The appeal to these frontline nurses is finally a national recognition of how important death with dignity is and the fact that something is being done to include all people, not just the lucky few in hospice. Action is being taken to support them in their nursing care and to support the dying and their families even more. The idea of each person being able to die with dignity and peace rather than struggle is paramount to them. They will be encouraged by and excited about *Golden Rooms* and will step forward to help make *Golden Rooms* a reality.

GERONTOLOGICAL NURSES

Gerontology has become a booming area of significance with the rapid aging of America. All areas related to the aging person's life are in need of rapid expansion and refinement, from housing to mobility to diet. Nowhere is this seen so dramatically as in the health care industry. Simply view the infomercials on television for mobility chairs and equipment, alternating pressure mattresses, and circulating enhancing devices. This alone is a huge industry.

The numbers of gerontological nurses are increasing, both those undergoing specific educational preparation and those simply drawn to working with the elderly. The National Gerontological Nursing Association (NGNA) has many thousands of members whose sole mission is to improve the quality of nursing care given to older adults. These nurses consciously or unconsciously are drawn to this place of caring service, and it is to these nurses that *Golden Rooms* will appeal.

NURSING ADMINISTRATORS

Nursing administrators are a rare breed walking between two worlds themselves—the world of administration and the world of nursing.

They deal with the practical application of quality nursing care while interfacing with the financial, political, and structural considerations. These nurses are critical to the actual implementation of *Golden Rooms* as they communicate with the outside world where they need to garner support and approval to build, remodel, or set aside a suite for the *Golden Rooms*. This is huge. These nurse executives will want to consider the cost savings of *Golden Rooms* for their institution; the draw of *Golden Rooms* for the general public; and the increased level of satisfaction of their customers, the patients, and their families.

The American Association of Nurse Executives (AONE) is the national organization of nurses who design, facilitate, and manage care. With more than 6,500 members, AONE is the voice of nursing leadership in health care. This impressive organization advances nursing practice and patient care, promotes nursing leadership excellence, and shapes public policy for health care (AONE).

Among the organizations' multiple coalitions there is one entitled Vision 2020 for nursing. This comprehensive declaration focuses on content that embraces end-of-life care:

> *The health of Americans is in serious jeopardy as the capacity of the nursing profession to care for an expanding, longer-living population continues to shrink. While nursing readily accepts the responsibility to fulfill its contract with society to maximize health, the profession's leadership recognizes that the current system of nursing practice, education and credentialing is inadequate to meet the future health care needs and demands of consumers. Transformation that realizes discrete scopes of practice and licensure, with clearly defined educational preparation for each scope of practice, is required. Inherent to this transformation is the requirement that nursing service leaders and nurse educators collaborate with delivery system stakeholders to design, refine and implement a nursing care system: one that facilitates the work of nursing in a satisfying and rewarding manner while promoting nursing advancement in clinical practice. (AONE, n.d.)*

CRITICAL CARE NURSES

A critical care unit is one of the most fast-paced, stressful places to work as a nurse. In the midst of all the technical equipment and stat orders is a person in need of physical, mental, emotional, and spiritual care. *Golden Rooms* where patients whose death is imminent in 3 to 10 days could be transferred would be very supportive for these nurses. They would relieve the nurses who could know that these special patients would be receiving nurturing holistic care and that their families would be there with them all the time, not just for minutes on the hour. Critical care nurses would appreciate their own workload being lessened, since the number of tests and procedures increases the nearer a patient is to death. They would have more time to attend to other patients and would experience almost a sense of relief. To be able to say to the patient, "Here, let me take off those leads and stop those machines; it's time to go to the *Golden Room*" would feel almost like a graduation . . . a coming release. The time of trying to heal the body has come to an end.

The American Association of Critical Care Nurses (AACN) has long been a leader in advocating quality, supportive end-of-life care. One of their three ongoing major advocacy initiatives has been attention to palliative end-of-life care. On their Web site (http://www.aacn.org/), they offer an e-learning course on palliative and end-of-life care. Using the complexity of symptom management and the trajectory of death, this course allows nurses to practice different approaches in a virtual environment. The AACN offers any number of courses and palliative care products.

Transfer from Acute or Nursing Home Care to the *Golden Room*

Most people are in acute care or a nursing home as they approach death. For this moment consider yourself there and reflect on the following questions. Where would you like to be during the hours or days preceding your passing from this physical plane? Pause now and conjure up the times and places that you remember when your loved ones and friends left this world. What was that like? Would you like the same for yourself? Or can you imagine being somewhere else? Do the exercise in Exhibit 12.1 for yourself. Once comfortable with your own parting, it will be much easier to lead those in your care on this same journey.

Take some moments to reflect on what you visualized and felt as you entered the *Golden Room*. Feel how your breathing has become gentle and relaxed. Note how the tension you are holding has lessened. Spend a few minutes enjoying this feeling before you continue.

When you are ready, complete the next exercise, in Exhibit 12.2, which focuses on the family and how they are feeling as they enter the *Golden Room* with their loved one. Certainly the family will also relax in the comfort of the *Golden Room*. As their stress is reduced they will be

EXHIBIT 12.1   Experience Your Entrance Into the
Golden Room

Envision the possibility that you are not feeling so well and some part of you recognizes that your time is about over. Engage your imagination as you contemplate the following scenario.

Feel the pressure of your body on the stretcher as you look up at the overhead lights as someone at the top of your head is pushing your bed forward. The lights glide by, one by one. Where are you going?

Imagine that you have reached this time and place. You are in an acute care setting or perhaps a nursing home. Rather than being transferred to the intensive care unit or the most distant room from the nurses' station, here's an idea of where you could go: The room you are going to on the stretcher is in a special cluster of rooms, either in an area of the hospital or nursing home or in a freestanding center. Each room is decorated with matching colors and contrasting accents from the theme of gold. One of the rooms is simpler with a tailored, classic décor. Another has rich damask drapes with a more opulent feel as well as an overstuffed, fold-out sleeping chair and richly covered walls. All the rooms have gold-painted or washable papered walls; they are softened with especially designed, sound-absorbent fabric-like material and windows with a view. Paintings depicting both distant landscape vistas and ethereal themes adorn the walls. Lamps with golden colored shades add to the sense that one is entering a beautiful, golden room.

As attendants move you off the stretcher, suddenly you are comfortable as you sink into flannel sheets and fluffed pillows. You are fully supported. As you gaze around this pretty room you notice a chaise lounge, a large overstuffed chair, a small bed across the room, and a little table and chairs. Why there is even a kitchenette with a microwave oven, a small refrigerator, and a sink as well as two bathrooms. It seems one is just for you and the other for your family and friends. There seems to be a draw curtain around both your bed and the other bed across the room, or maybe you are even in a private room. Looks like plenty of space in here.

You feel so much better with the subclavian intravenous line detached. Now that you are more aware, you notice that even that irritating burning from the insertion site is gone. All that is left is a small "port a catheter" on the inside of your wrist. The nurse tells you that this serves as an injection or infusion site should you need any special medications or fluid. Suddenly it's trouble-free again to turn from side to side without the tangle of all the tubes, and getting out of bed will be easier with the small lift right beside the bed. Perhaps they can hoist you into that nice straightbacked chair you see next to the bed.

The bed feels so good, except you still note that slight crinkle under the flannel sheet that indicates there is a plastic protector between the sheet and the mattress, but it is not as noticeable with the soft flannel sheet as it was with the cotton ones. You sink in and better assess your surroundings. Why there are your daughter and son-in-law; how nice to see them again. And who is that little girl with them? She certainly looks familiar—could that be Patty, their daughter, my granddaughter? Oh my, I feel mixed up, but it is nice to see familiar faces here. Now what is that little girl doing climbing up beside me in the bed? Oh well, she seems sweet, and it is nice to have someone holding my hand.

EXHIBIT 12.2   Experience the Family's Entrance Into the *Golden Room*

You or your dying loved one slips into unconsciousness and/or a deep sleep. The family gets comfortable in the extra furnishings and turns on the television. What, no news programs or game shows? What appears is a channel selection of nature scenes accompanied by lovely music. You are immediately lulled into a calm state, very different from what you felt as you agreed to move your relative to the *Golden Room*. Remember how frazzled you were just yesterday? Making the decision was difficult, but right now everything seems much easier. Then your loved one was hooked up to the IV, a subclavian line, the cardiac monitor, and, oxygen tubing. Now he or she is sleeping. Think of yourself being there—I am stretched out on the chaise lounge; Patty is getting some orange juice from the refrigerator. She's even pouring me some. I rub my temples and stretch back in the lounge chair as Patty gets on the bed and my spouse sinks into the big easy chair. Okay, this is better, I tell myself.

EXHIBIT 12.2   (*Continued*)

The next day the nurse offers a plethora of options. For example, would I like a back massage, reflexology, healing touch, chakra balancing, or Reiki? To help the family and the patient decide, a guidebook is available that describes the numerous complementary therapies offered here. The nurse reviews options to help choose the most appropriate ones for this patient in this setting. Apparently you can choose whatever you want for the patient and for an additional fee even select one of the therapies for yourself.

better able to be in the moment with their loved one and better able to cope on all levels with this final journey.

As an aside: Did you actually do these two exercises? Or did you quickly read through them with the idea "let's see where this is going" or "I'll do them later." If you did not do the exercises, you were so busy getting to the future that you were not in the moment. Go back and take the time to be in the moment. This is a small example of how we miss being here because our mind is busy trying to get to the next thing to do.

NURSING HOME DIRECTORS

How fortunate we are to have these nurses who also walk between the two worlds. Nursing home directors are very familiar with death and dying since few people get out of nursing homes alive, and if they do, they eventually come back. Nursing home directors are familiar with transfers to the hospital for emergency care and transfers back to the home. It will be incredible when these nurses realize how advantageous it is to have *Golden Room* suites in their nursing homes or to be able to transfer patients to *Golden Room* centers. Either way they are in a win–win situation because the family can be assured that if they cannot be there, their loved one will be cared for by specially trained health care professionals and attended to with honor and love. And if the family is absent, their loved one will not die alone. This is an added perk for a nursing home. As families begin to experience *Golden Rooms*, they will begin to look for facilities that either have suites in house or are connected to a freestanding center.

Transfer from Nursing Homes to the *Golden Room*

Transfer from the nursing home to the *Golden Room* can be a similar experience for the patient and the family to the one you experienced earlier. It is a time of releasing the struggle, the excess baggage of the remaining tubes and machines, and being in a place of gentle love and peace. It feels almost exciting that the end is near—the journey of 1,000 steps is finally nearing completion. It is a bittersweet experience for the family and yet for their loved one a welcome release.

EDUCATORS AND RESEARCHERS

Both educators and researchers will appreciate the underlying significance of the *Golden Room* and the creation of a place for a dignified release from this physical plane. Educators will value the opportunity to spend more time on the importance of nurses' self-care as they help students explore their feelings and beliefs about death and dying. *Golden Rooms* are an almost perfect example of nursing care at its finest because all levels of care are provided—physical, mental, emotional, and spiritual. Researchers have already been studying the end of life and spirituality. Here is the opportunity to do advanced research on a select group of health care professionals in a select location at one of the least understood moments in life. Here is the prospect of learning more about how to support nurses in doing what they love to do and being present with the loved one and the family at the end of life. Such research has the potential to recognize and improve the necessary self-care that nurses require in order to not numb out in a profession that asks for giving of the self from the heart as well as the hands.

PROFESSIONAL PREPARATION CORE COMPONENTS: END-OF-LIFE CARE

As with any area of nursing care, careful consideration needs to be given to the criteria for the health care providers for the *Golden Room*. Most nurses come equipped with some understanding of palliative care, which over time often becomes the last thing that is considered after all the treatments and medications. To work in the *Golden Room* all health care providers will need to have both initial and ongoing education in holistic palliative care and comfort measures and in holistic self-care.

EXHIBIT 12.3   National Board for Certification of Hospice and Palliative Nurses Certifications

* Advanced Certified Hospice and Palliative Nurse (ACHPN)
* Certified Hospice and Palliative Nurse (CHPN)
* Certified Hospice and Palliative Licensed Nurse (CHPLN)
* Certified Hospice and Palliative Nursing Assistant (CHPNA)
* Certified Hospice and Palliative Care Administrator (CHPCA)

From *National Board for Certification of Hospice and Palliative Nurses* (2010).

Certification is the educational track most recognized as the route to expert knowledge. It is the formal recognition of specialized knowledge, skills, and experience. A certification credential after your name demonstrates to the profession a high level of commitment to your field of practice and a high level of knowledge and skill unique to your role. Specialty certification enhances the professional reputation of nurse leaders and practitioners. A number of specialty organizations offer certification programs. Palliative care certification is offered by one of these organizations. Since the *Golden Room* is an extension of this principle it follows that nurses interested in the *Golden Room* concept would build on this already strong foundation.

The only organization offering certification on all four levels of palliative and hospice nursing care is the National Board for Certification of Hospice and Palliative Nurses (NBCHPN). Certification is valid for a 4-year period and is renewable. There are over 16,000 health care professional certified by NBCHPN (2010). At this time NBCHPN offers five area of certification, as seen in Exhibit 12.3.

To be eligible for the NBCHPN® examination, an applicant must hold a current, unrestricted nurse license in the United States, its territories, or the equivalent in Canada. NBCHPN® recommends that candidates have at least 2 years of experience in hospice and palliative nursing practice to consider themselves eligible for certification as a Certified Hospice and Palliative Nurse (CHPN®). Candidates that sit for and pass the RN certification exam are granted the CHPN® credential (Certified Hospice and Palliative Nurse). (www.nbchpn.org/Displayaspx? Title=RNoverview)

The seven general components of the registered nurse certification are presented in Exhibit 12.4. Notice that 66% of the components are

EXHIBIT 12.4   **Seven Components of Registered Nurse Certification in Hospice and Palliative Care**

• Patient care: Life-limiting conditions in adult patients	14%
• Patient care: Pain management	25%
• Patient care: Symptom management	27%
• Care of patient and family	11%
• Education and advocacy	9%
• Interdisciplinary/collaborative practice	8%
• Professional issues (practice and professional development)	6%

From *Hospice and Palliative Care Certification* (n.d.).

focused on the patients with 11% focused on the patients and their families. Professional issues—both practice and professional development—comprise 6%. There is no reference to or consideration of holistic self-care for the nursing professional.

The NGNA also certifies nurses. This association offers a two-day certification preparation course annually prior to the start of its annual convention. An online certification review course for the generalist gerontological nursing certification is available through one of the links on their Web site (http://www.ngna.org/). This generalist certification is the basic preparation for working in the *Golden Room* and is required for all registered nurses. The certification for the other staff and administration is also required for them to work in the *Golden Room*. Here we are focusing on the registered nurse (Exhibit 12.5).

Additional Criteria and Certification for the *Golden Room*

Registered nurses must hold a bachelor's degree in nursing. *The Golden Room* certification program is divided into three levels and includes areas that are not included in the hospice and palliative care program. Table 12.1 gives the title of each level and the number of hours of training required for each. The first two levels are required to work in the *Golden Room*. Level I must be taken prior to beginning employment. Level I content is outlined in Exhibit 12.6 and includes areas with more specific holistic content than in the CHPN credential as well as additional areas and insights.

EXHIBIT 12.5   Research Perspective

The first known study considering the correlation between certified nurses and patient care was conducted in 2000 by the Nursing Credentialing Research Coalition. Many positive outcomes brought about through care by certified nurses were identified; these include

- Increased patient satisfaction ratings
- Decreased patient adverse events
- Improved communication and collaboration with other providers
- Decreased disciplinary events
- Fewer work-related injuries
- Increases in both personal growth and professional satisfaction

Other studies of the certified workforce followed and provided preliminary indications that certification furnishes nurses with the ability to improve outcomes in nursing care. Findings also confirmed that certification adds to retention of staff, improves patient outcomes, and promotes greater efficiency. Patient care and safety are significantly affected by certification, and the specialized knowledge and skills needed to provide high-quality and safe care are definitely produced by specialty certification. Certification is a very powerful marketing tool that creates a high level of support and respect.

From *Hospice and Palliative Care Certification* (n.d.).

Level II is must be completed within 6 months of employment. Level II content is outlined in Exhibit 12.7 and includes information about self-care and being in the present moment. Level III is required for teaching in the *Golden Room* Certificate Program. The content is yet to be determined. Nurses may be grandfathered into this certifica-

TABLE 12.1   *The Golden Room* Certification by Level and Number of Hours

Level I: Introduction to the *Golden Room*	30 hours
Level II: Introduction to Self-Care	30 hours
Level III: Teaching Certification	30 hours

EXHIBIT 12.6   Level I: Introduction to the *Golden Room* Nursing Content

- Palliative care for the dying person
- Holistic care for the dying person
- Living well/dying well
- Pain management
- The dying person as teacher
- Rituals: personal, family, ethnic, religious
- Family and friends
- The language of dying: verbal and nonverbal
- Complementary therapies

EXHIBIT 12.7   Level II: Introduction to Self-Care Nursing Content

- Diet
- Exercise and movement
- Sleep
- Hydration
- Meditation/relaxation
- Breathing exercises
- Reflective practice
- Journaling
- Self-reflection
- Self-assessment
- Humor, laughter, and play

tion at a specified dated if they met specific requirements that have yet to be determined.

Continuing Education for Maintaining *Golden Room* Certification

To maintain their certification, nurses will be required to obtain 10 hours of ongoing education every 2 years in any area surrounding palliative care, death and dying, and self-care. These programs are being proposed now.

SELF-CARE

At the heart of the *Golden Room* is the understanding that in order to take care of the dying and their families, nurses must first and foremost take care of themselves. The following gives an explanation of burnout and sample scripts to assist nurses in maintaining their balance and clarity while working with the dying and their families.

Burnout is a common factor in the health care professions and certainly one that needs to be addressed in advance so that the health care providers who truly love and enjoy what they do also receive the benefit of goodness, compassion, peace, dignity, and release—in this case, release of stress. Meditation is one technique used to assist in balancing and releasing the stresses of one's life. Meditation has many connotations, from sitting in a certain position to being quiet in nature to sitting in a favorite quiet spot in one's home. It can also be thought of as reflective contemplation where by one turns one's attention from the normal activity of the mind inward into the still, quiet recesses. Many can do this with practice through a breath or two, but there are also simple yet effective ways to bring this about. This is a skill that has been effectively used over the years. One of these is a type of progressive relaxation as described in Exhibit 12.8. This can easily take 10 to 15 minutes.

EXHIBIT 12.8   Progressive Relaxation Script

As you close your eyes become aware of your breathing . . . notice its pattern and rate . . . nothing to change, simply notice . . . move your attention to your toes and simply focus your attention here . . . gently stay with your breathing . . . move your attention to the calves of your legs . . . stay with your breathing . . . to your hips . . . so gently, nothing to do here but be aware . . . to your lower belly . . . notice your stomach area . . . stay with your breathing . . . gently, easily . . . move your attention to your chest and lungs . . . notice the rise and fall of the chest . . . simply notice ... stay with your breath . . . move your attention to your face . . . your chin . . . your ears . . . your eyes . . . your forehead . . . and the top of your head . . . and return to your breath . . . simply step back and notice your entire body all at once . . . gently easily . . . stay with your breath . . . feel the rise and fall of your chest . . . become aware of the room around you and when you are ready open your eyes.

Nurses are encouraged to practice this at home daily during Level II certification.

Stepping back into that still, quiet place is very beneficial for clarity of thinking and action. Often the health care professional does need to move in the moment and does not have the time to do a longer meditation, so shorter ones are also extremely beneficial. An example of one is given in Exhibit 12.9. For those emergency times when you are racing down the hall toward a patient's room, a even faster, simple script as described in Exhibit 12.10 could be used.

EXHIBIT 12.9   Script for Short Relaxation

STOP! Take five slow, deep breaths, feeling the cool air as it enters your nostrils and the warm air as it leaves the nostrils. Put your entire attention on your breathing and the feelings it produces in your body. Return to your work with a still mind and ready to take action from a balanced inner space.

EXHIBIT 12.10   Script for Emergency Situations

As you are moving toward the emergency
become aware of your steps and
feel the change of weight from the heel to the toe
with each step . . .
Spend your time here in the present moment walking.
You will know exactly what to do when you arrive.
When you arrive,
STOP momentarily,
take a deep breath,
and
walk into the room,
refreshed,
in the moment,
and
clear of mind.

The more nurses learn to be in the present moment, the more energetic they are, the more clear, the more decisive, the more openhearted, the more alert. The quality of nursing care goes up exponentially. Working first with the nurse, who in turn works with the dying person and the family, enables everyone to shift to a wider place in consciousness. Thereby the nurse is able to fully assist and be present in the moment for the person to experience this last, most sacred time of his or her life, moving through the portal to infinity.

SUMMARY

The multidimensional structure of support, education, and concern needed to implement end-of-life care through *Golden Rooms* is already in place. The key lies in mobilizing, and here is where the nursing profession shines. Nurses on all levels know how to activate and organize to ensure quality care for their patients. Now the patient becomes an idea whose time has come to be implemented in diverse and meaningful ways. This action surrounds a fundamental shift in consciousness around death and dying to one of dignity and openness. This is a noble task, one coming from deeper wisdom. Nurses are known for taking on responsibilities that bring relief to their patients and, historically, have gone and will go to any length. As our consciousness changes and, as nurses, we accept the deep inner knowing of death with dignity that we desire for all people, this transformation will occur with an increasing intensity. Like the 100th-monkey phenomena this shift in consciousness requires a critical mass, and it will automatically become the expectation rather than the exception in the dying process. Here at the beginning of the 21st century is the time to start a movement to change the quality of dying in America to one of dignity and comfort that is available to everyone. Now is the time to focus on *Golden Rooms*.

Words of Wisdom

Perhaps the only limits to the human mind are those we believe in.

—Willis Harmon

REFERENCES

Hospice and Palliative Care Certification. (n.d.). Retrieved May 6, 2010, from http://www.nbchpn.org/DisplayPage.aspx?Title=Candidate Handbook and Application

National Board for Certification of Hospice and Palliative Nurses. (2010). Retrieved May 5, 2010, from http://www.nbchpn.org/

American Association of Nurse Executives. http://www.aone.org/

American Association of Nurse Executives. "Vision 2020 for Nursing." Retrieved fromhttp://www.aone.org/aone/advocacy/npec.html

13 *Creating a Plan or Proposal*

There is nothing more difficult to take in hand, more perilous to conduct, or more uncertain in its success, than to take the lead in the introduction of a new order of things because the innovator has for enemies all those who have done well under the old conditions, and lukewarm defenders in those who may do well under the new.
—Machiavelli

*R*ACHEL'S STORY   *Several years ago I was invited to give a talk about my work with people with cancer to a group of women physicians at a local meeting of the American Women's Medical Association. In the discussion after the talk, an internist commented that she would find this work difficult. She had avoided caring for people with cancer because a certain percentage of them die and she found it upsetting to care for dying patients. "I hate it when I've run out of treatments, when there is nothing more I can do," she confessed. Others in the group nodded their agreement.*

I asked them when they first became uncomfortable with these situations. The women were surprised to notice that they had not been as uncomfortable before medical school. As the discussion went on, it became clearer that we were more uncomfortable in these situations as doctors than as women. As women, we knew there was something simple and natural in just being there together. Slowly some insights emerged. Women have always been present at these times, at death and birth and in many of the other transitions, as comforters and companions, as witnesses, to mark the importance of the moment.

One of the physicians talked about caring for her dying mother when she was nineteen years old. She had expected a great deal less of herself then. At first she had driven her mother to her doctor's appointments, shopped for food, and run errands. As her mother grew weaker, she had prepared tempting meals and cleaned the house. When her mother stopped eating, she had listened to her and read to her for hours. When her mother slipped into coma, she had changed her sheets, bathed her, and rubbed her back with lotion.

There always seemed to be something more to do, a way to care. These ways became simpler and simpler. "In the end," she told us, "I just held her and sang."

There was a long thoughtful silence. Then one of the older women said that she too had tended to avoid situations when there were no treatments left. She had felt powerless. But she saw now that even when there was nothing left to do medically, there were still other things she could say or do that might matter, maybe just kind words. Ways she could still be of help. She had simply forgotten. Her voice wavered slightly. I looked at her more closely. This tough and competent sixty-year-old surgeon had tears in her eyes. It was quite amazing. (Remen, 2006, pp 44–45)

REFLECTIONS ON ISSUES OF CONCERN

1. What have we lost in our fast-paced technological and medical treatments? How do we recapture it?
2. Even health care professionals can "run out of things to do." When is it time to stop and honor the natural cycle of life? Who gets to decide?
3. As a nurse what is one thing that you can change in your nursing practice right now that will assist the honoring of the life cycle?
4. What are the guiding principles for your life? For your practice? Have you ever compromised these? For what end? Was it worth it? How did you feel?
5. Perhaps it is time to practice goodness, compassion, peace, dignity, and release in all aspects of our life. What would be the consequences?
6. Of the numerous nursing diagnoses, which one or two do you find most related to your nursing care with end-of-life patients?
7. Are there any prototypes of *Golden Rooms* already in existence where you live? Have you checked them out? Would you please contact the authors and share them?
8. Engaging and building support begins with small steps and can go far. What are three things that you are willing to do to build consensus and take action?

THE NEED FOR CONSENSUS AND ACTION

On March 22, 2010, the U.S. Congress passed a comprehensive health care reform bill that among other things was projected to provide health insurance to approximately 95% of U.S. citizens. Heralded as a long-awaited step in health care reform, prototypes of this bill had been discussed and proposed since the Roosevelt era. Times are certainly changing and health care is changing along with the times. This time of incredible revamping of the payment system for health care is the exact time when consensus and action are needed both to implement the *Golden Room* and to change the consciousness around death and dying. Reading this book certainly puts all the facts and figures in one place. A tacit agreement has been identified as to the need for an option for death with dignity that is available for all dying persons. It is time to take action and move into solutions. It is time for implementing the *Golden Room*.

GUIDING PRINCIPLES

As medical professionals our first and primary guiding principle is to do no harm and, as we do this, assist each dying person and his or her family to experience this last journey with dignity and as much ease as possible. As we come together at this momentous time of great change and transition, it is time to let go of the need to prove anything. It is a time for all health care per-sonnel to let go of their own biases and come to this dying person and family in love and gentle being. It is a time to forgo further end-of-life medical treatment and instead be of comfort physically, mentally, emotionally, and spiritually. There really is always something to do, and as you recognize this, it becomes simpler and eas-ier. There definitely are ways to care. The sacredness in this time of tran-sition is like no other and invites a reciprocal response from each person present, especially the health care personnel.

The second principle is based on the Law of the Six Nations, the Iro-quois Confederacy, which simply states, "In all our deliberations we must be mindful of the impact of our decisions on the seven generations to follow ours." We, like the Iroquois people, must initiate a place, a criterion, an educational process for nurses, and a return to a conscious-ness that honors and assists all dying people to end life with goodness, compassion, peace, dignity, and release.

Our third guiding principle is to remember that what we place our in-tention and attention on becomes our reality. As our consciousness shifts into greater awareness of the simple, more humane ways to live and the honoring of all living things, it becomes apparent that these *Golden Room* centers are urgently needed. The change begins in consciousness as people become deeply moved by the need for a new and innovative perspective on death and dying. Having felt this shift in consciousness, we wrote this book to light the way and call forth these deep inner qualities in you, the nurse, the reader. As this awareness grows the natural organic outcome is that the people, the resources, and the means of support appear. This sounds like magic to the mind, but the deeper realization is that what we put our attention on is what appears in our life. When we follow our deep inner heart feelings, the opportunities present themselves. Our first step, then, is spreading the word through written and verbal media.

Although these three guiding principles appear on the surface to be simple and straightforward, they require constant vigilance to keep them in front of all those who move to take action to bring *Golden Rooms* into reality. This means not compromising our values for the sake of expediency or putting the idea into a committee for further consideration. It simply means building consensus, taking action, and moving forward. We have made the commitment to move forward. Who will join us? The time has come to step up and take a stand for what is right. The time has come for the *Golden Room*.

RESOURCES

Incredible resources are at our disposal in the 21st century. Our natural resources for fostering end-of-life care include individuals, organizations, publications, media, and numerous aspects of the Internet. Communication through all of our resources helps us to link to and create changes in the world. Using our resources provides us opportunities to spread the word about *Golden Rooms* and death with dignity. The health care reform movement is gaining momentum, and certainly the *Golden Room* greatly addresses reform and improving the quality of life . . . and death. The health care industry and insurance companies are searching for cost-containing and cost-saving methods of doing things.

Individuals

Nurses are at the forefront of health care reform and have been from the very beginning. Florence Nightingale knew and experienced what it takes to improve health care conditions in hospitals. Now it is our turn to pick up the baton and continue the efforts to improve end-of-life care for everyone. Nurses are our greatest resource for both change and support.

Organizations

Nursing is gifted with literally hundreds of organizations. Many are oriented to the end of life. Associations such as the Gerontological Nursing Society, the Palliative and Hospice Organization, and the American Association of Critical Care Nurses are all examples of organizations that seek to improve the end of life. To recall how we can be strong in numbers, we can remember the old adage that the whole is greater than the sum of the parts. Just think of the resource power of our nursing organizations.

Publications

Ever read a nursing journal, news magazine, or a newspaper? Of course you have, and you likely do so on a regular basis. Consider the depth and scope of knowledge generated and communicated through our scholarly publications and then extrapolate that to the popular press. Then realize how broadly we can disseminate information to others through our writing and publications.

Media

Media include such things as audio recordings, videos, PowerPoint offerings, radio programs, television, and even movies. Nurses are becoming increasingly present in media productions, not only developing them but also starring in them. Consider our resource power when we utilize media.

Internet

All the numerous dimensions of the Internet are staggering. There are personal and organization Web addresses, links, blogs, Facebook pages, email, chat rooms, and so on. We have at our disposal the most innovative communication tool in the history of humankind. If we can collectively come to believe and accept that our kindred *Homo sapiens* deserve a good death, a dignified death, the best possible death, then consider how rapidly we can spread the word.

ALIGNING CARE PLANS TO GOALS
AND CIRCUMSTANCES

Personalization of nursing care is very important for each dying patient and his or her family. Many nurses use the holistic caring process to focus on the care of the whole unique person to respect and advocate for the person's rights and choices. "Based on holistic assessment and identification of the person's health patterns, decisions about care flow from collaboration with the person, other healthcare providers, and significant others" (Potter & Frisch, 2009, p. 146). This holistic caring process utilizes a model that is good for use with a dying patient and includes assessment; patterns, problems, and needs; and outcomes.

During each step in the care plan consider using this process. For example, during assessment consider intuitive thinking along with other hard data. During the phase of identifying patterns, challenges, needs, consider the diagnostic statement, levels of care and prevention, and nursing diagnosis as a descriptive tool. Outcome identification will lead to the development of a therapeutic care plan. In this final phase the nurse develops a plan that identifies strategies and alternatives to attain the desired outcomes. Naturally, following the implementation of this process, the nurse evaluates the plan. Then finally ask yourself whether progress was made toward attainment of outcomes while recognizing and honoring the nature of the goals.

NURSING DIAGNOSES RELATIVE
TO END-OF-LIFE CARE

A wide range of issues important in end-of-life care are currently reflected well by nursing diagnoses. Among the most pertinent are spirituality, coping, anxiety, grieving, and a host of symptom management issues such as self-care deficits, pain, and dyspnea. As we continue to refine and redefine our diagnoses, this crucial life stage must not be missed (Carroll-Johnson, 2001). Nursing care at the end of life in the *Golden Room* involves mainly palliative care encompassing both the person and the family. The North American Nursing Diagnosis Association (NANDA) classifies and categorizes nursing diagnoses for every aspect of a patient's condition. Many of these diagnoses are germane to end-of-life nursing care. Potential nursing diagnoses in Table 13.1 are suggested and are not exhaustive but rather open to refinement in specific situations.

TABLE 13.1   Nursing Diagnoses for the End of Life

Comfort measures	
Pain management	
Ego integrity	• May exhibit stress related to recent changes in ability to care for self and decision to accept hospice services • Feelings of helplessness/hopelessness, sorrow, anger; choked feeling • Fear of the dying process, loss of physical and/or mental abilities • Concern about impact of death on significant other/family • Inner conflict about beliefs, meaning of life/death • Financial concerns; lack of preparation (e.g., will, power of attorney, funeral) • May exhibit deep sadness, crying, anxiety, apathy • Altered communication patterns, social isolation, withdrawal
Social interaction	• May report apprehension about caregiver's ability to provide care • Changes in family roles/usual patterns of responsibility • May exhibit difficulty adapting to changes imposed by condition/dying process

From "Nursing Care Plans End of Life/Hospice Care." http://nursingcareplan.blogspot.com/2007/02/ncp-end-of-life-hospice-care.html

Diagnosis centers around symptom and pain management and psychological, spiritual, and grief support. The main nursing priorities are listed in Exhibit 13.1. Note the seeming simplicity of the nursing care priorities, but do not be fooled. These priorities require a shift in consciousness to be effective so that the compassion and dignity are felt by the dying person and the family.

Studies of Application of Nursing Diagnoses

There are a number of ongoing NANDA (North American Nursing Diagnosis Association) application studies. An international team conducted a content validation study for the elements of the nursing diagnosis Impaired Memory and included aging as a related factor. The definition, defining characteristics, and related factors of NANDA-I

EXHIBIT 13.1   Nursing Priorities at the End of Life

1. Control pain.
2. Prevent/manage complications.
3. Maintain quality of life as much as possible.
4. Have plans in place to meet patient's/family's last wishes (e.g., care setting, advance directives, will, funeral).

From "Nursing Care Plans End of Life/Hospice Care." http://nursingcareplan.blog spot.com/2007/02/ncp-end-of-life-hospice-care.html

were evaluated by experts, as was the proposed related factor "aging." Elements of the NANDA-I diagnosis Impaired Memory and the proposed related factor of aging were validated in this country's Brazilian context and suggest that the NANDA-I diagnoses should be tested and validated in the elderly, in order to take their specific needs into account, thus contributing to quality nursing care for these patients (Chaves, de Barros, & Marini, 2010). We can extrapolate from this study to suggest that NANDA diagnoses can also be more frequently used with patients at the end of life.

One team did a comprehensive, systematic review of the outcomes of nursing diagnostics. It examined effects on the quality of documentation of assessment; frequency, accuracy, and completeness of nursing diagnoses; and coherence between nursing diagnoses, interventions, and outcomes. The researchers found that use of nursing diagnoses improved the quality of documented patient assessments, identification of commonly occurring diagnoses within similar settings, and coherence among nursing diagnoses, interventions, and outcomes. The trend indicated that nursing diagnostics improved assessment documentation, the quality of interventions reported, and outcomes attained (Muller-Staub, Lavin, Needham, & van Achterberg, 2006).

A U.S. study described a customized electronic medical record documentation system, called Epic, that provides an electronic health record, using standardized taxonomies for nursing documentation. Nurses used standardized nursing nomenclature including NANDA-I diagnoses, nursing interventions classification, and nursing outcomes classification in a measurable and user-friendly format using the care plan activity. They found that the key factors in the success of the project included close collaboration among staff nurses and information technology staff, ongoing support and encouragement from the vice president/

chief nursing officer, the ready availability of expert resources, and nursing ownership of the project. Use of this evidence-based documentation enhanced institutional leadership in clinical documentation (Klehr, Hafner, Spelz, Steen, & Weaver, 2009).

A Swiss researcher found that carefully implementing classifications led to enhanced, accurately stated nursing diagnoses, more effective nursing interventions, and better patient outcomes. Based on the results of this study, the inclusion of NANDA international diagnoses with related interventions and outcomes in electronic health records is suggested (Müller-Staub, 2009). Since electronic medical records are the wave of the future, it makes sense to consider incorporating nursing diagnoses, interventions, and outcomes into the records of our end-of-life patients.

NANDA strives to ensure that end-of-life concerns are named and reflected in appropriate nursing diagnoses. Complementing the diagnoses are appropriate nursing interventions and nursing outcomes. With a concerted effort all formerly accepted diagnoses, as well as those under consideration and yet-to-be-developed diagnostic labels, should be scrutinized to ascertain that, if appropriate, the end of life is reflected in the definitions, related factors, and defining characteristics. Validation of a diagnosis must not be considered complete unless end-of-life concerns are incorporated (Carroll-Johnson, 2001).

PROTOTYPES ALREADY IN EXISTENCE

The primary prototypes that serve as the setting for dying in America are hospitals, nursing homes, an occasional freestanding hospice, or the person's own home. Each setting is useful and works in some circumstances but not all. Without preplanning it is sometimes difficult to transport between settings, and differently prepared personnel often have conflicting expectations as to appropriate outcomes.

Hospitals

Many deaths occur in hospitals. Most people receive some hospital care during the process of diagnosis or after being diagnosed with a serious or terminal condition. Since curing disease and prolonging life are the primary missions of hospitals, this is generally not the place to be during one's last days. In addition, hospital culture and the caregivers who work there often regard death as a failure. Modern medicine shines in the hospital where the mission is rescuing, stabilizing, and curing people with serious physical problems, but is this the place to die?

Nursing Homes

The vast majority of people die in nursing homes. The care they receive there varies greatly from one home to another and from one geographic region to another. Some homes are small with a stable staff; others are chains with ever-changing personnel. Some are certified by both Medicare and Medicaid, and others are not. Even within one agency care may differ from one wing to another depending on staffing level and the personality of the primary caregiver (vocational nurse or aide) working the shift when the death actually occurs.

For some patients coming to a nursing home, death is expected soon, and that is why they are admitted. Others may spend years there before their final decline. Most who enter a nursing home and stay for more than a few months will die there or soon be transferred to a hospital. Few will ever return to their home again.

Hospice Care

There are two basic types of hospice care: inpatient and home.

Inpatient

Within this category are respite inpatient care and general patient care. To receive respite care the patient moves to a nursing home or some other inpatient facility to order to give in-home caregivers a respite from the physical and emotional tolls of end-of-life care. For general care the patient receives hospice care in an inpatient facility for management of acute needs.

Hospice Home Care

Within this category there are two types of service: routine home care or continuous home care. Hospice caregivers provide a full scope of services in the patient's home. During continuous home care more intensive care is provided, often with skilled nursing care for 8 out of 24 hours of the day. Acute symptom management prevents the need for hospitalization (Editor, 2007).

Home Care

Some people still die at home without outside care. For the most part, they either do not qualify for inpatient or hospice programs, or they are not perceived to be dying either by themselves or by others. The problem with this choice for the end of life—or the lack of recognition that they are terminal—is that by the time they or family members realize they are at the end of life, they may be in acute pain and are then rushed by ambulance to the hospital. The emergency department is not the place to be in the final stages of life. Consequently we must encourage those in their final weeks or life to make a conscious choice for end-of-life care and consequently ease a suffering and/or solitary death (Exhibit 13.2).

ENGAGING AND BUILDING SUPPORT

Awareness and a sense of urgency to move forward with *Golden Rooms* are critical at this juncture. Already the first subtle steps have been taken, with critical attention to a strategy of networking and advancing consensus and support in ever-larger circles. Certainly the following areas

EXHIBIT 13.2   Point of View

End-of-life care is a wonderful opportunity for nursing to demonstrate its best face. Clearly nurses are the health care professionals who are most willing to be present and best able to articulate what dying patients most need. Less clear are the strategies necessary to ensure that nurses have the time necessary to attend to the care needs of the dying person. I have to believe that an important first step in calling attention to the need for increased nursing presence is our ability to name and measure what we do and why we do it. The precision with which we describe this care can help determine and drive the ability to provide what is needed to all patients.

From Carroll-Johnson (2001).

are critical to the success of *Golden Rooms*, and more areas of support will open up in the process.

Government and Legislative Support

Information on how to contact state and federal representatives is easily located on the Internet at http://www.congress.org/. This Web site provides one foundation for effective grassroots advocacy. There are tips on telephoning, writing, and emailing elected officials as well as explanations of the commonly used titles of the congressional staff that assist members of Congress during their terms in office. Knowing titles and principal functions assists in professional communication. A locator is available to contact state elected officials across the country.

Professional Organization Support

Support for the end of life is available from multiple professional organizations. A few are highlighted here.

American Academy of Hospice and Palliative Medicine

The American Academy of Hospice and Palliative Medicine is an organization of physicians and other medical professionals dedicated to excellence in palliative medicine and the prevention and relief of suffering among patients and families by providing education and clinical practice standards, fostering research, facilitating personal and professional development of its members, and advocating changes in public policy (http://www.aahpm.org).

Association for Death Education and Counseling

The Association for Death Education and Counseling (ADEC) is one of the oldest interdisciplinary organizations in the field of dying, death, and bereavement. Its nearly 2,000 members include a wide array of mental and medical health personnel, educators, clergy, funeral directors, and volunteers (http://www.adec.org).

Compassionate Friends

The mission of the Compassionate Friends is to help families move toward the positive resolution of grief following the death of a child of any age and to provide information to help others be supportive (http://www.compassionatefriends.org).

Nursing Organizations

Nursing has a plethora of organizations that have a vested interest in end-of-life issues. Each is a terrific resource to garner support for Golden Rooms. A select sample follows.

Hospice and Palliative Nurses Association

The Hospice and Palliative Nurses Association (HPNA) is a distinctive membership organization with individual nurse membership levels for the advanced practitioner, generalist nurse, licensed practical nurse, Vocational nurse, nursing assistant, and associate (nonnursing). The expertise of these nurses puts them in a unique place of authority for specialty nursing resources, direction, and information. They sustain and support the nursing team's compassionate work with the dying person and his or her family as they journey together through the experience of life-limiting illness.

HPNA is the collaborative and visionary professional hospice and palliative specialty nursing organization with evidence-based educational tools to assist members of the nursing team with

- Ensuring quality nursing care delivery
- Managing complex symptoms along with grief and bereavement
- Supporting one another and nurturing future leaders through networking and mentoring
- Having the difficult conversations
- Educating health care providers and family about the hospice or palliative care philosophy
- Influencing palliative nursing through leadership and research (http://www.hpna.org)

American Association of Critical-Care Nurses

The American Association of Critical-Care Nurses (AACN) has established an end-of-life leadership consortium and designed an agenda for the nursing profession on end-of-life care. They have yearly weekend certificate training for palliative end-of-life care (http://www.aacn.org/WD/Practice/Docs/Designing_Agenda.pdf).

American Association of Colleges of Nursing

The American Association of Colleges of Nursing (AACN) is the national voice for America's baccalaureate- and higher-degree nursing education programs. AACN's educational, research, governmental advocacy, data collection, publication, and other programs work to establish quality standards for bachelor's and graduate-degree nursing education; assist deans and directors in implementing those standards; influence the nursing profession to improve health care; and promote public support of baccalaureate and graduate education, research, and practice in nursing—the nation's largest health care profession. AACN's End of Life Nursing Education Consortium (ELNED) holds yearly palliative care training programs across the United States (http://www.aacn. nche.edu/index.htm).

American Academy of Nursing

The American Academy of Nursing (AAN) is an organization of distinguished leaders in nursing who have been recognized for their outstanding contributions to the profession and to health care. The academy, established in 1973 under the aegis of the American Nurses Association, is constituted to provide visionary leadership to the nursing profession and the public in shaping future health policy, advancing scientific knowledge, and influencing the development of effective health care policies and practices (http://www.aanet.org/).

American College of Nurse Practitioners

Founded in 1993, the American College of Nurse Practitioners (ACNP) is a national nonprofit membership organization headquartered in Washington, DC. The ACNP is focused on advocacy and keeping nurse practitioners current on legislative, regulatory, and clinical practice issues that affect them in the rapidly changing health care arena (http:// www.acnpweb.org/).

American Nurses Association

The American Nurses Association is a full-service professional organization representing the nation's 2.6 million registered nurses through its 54 constituent state associations and 13 organizational affiliate members (http://www.ana.org/).

American Organization of Nurse Executives

Founded in 1967, the American Organization of Nurse Executives, a subsidiary of the American Hospital Association, is a national organization of nearly 4,000 nurses who design, facilitate, and manage care. Its mission is to represent nurse leaders who improve health care (http://www.aone.org/).

Emergency Nurses Association

The Emergency Nurses Association (ENA) is the national association for professional nurses dedicated to the advancement of emergency nursing practice (http://www.ena.org/).

National Council of State Boards of Nursing

The National Council of State Boards of Nursing (NCSBN) is a not-for-profit organization whose purpose is to provide an organization through which boards of nursing act and counsel together on matters of common interest and concern affecting the public health, safety, and welfare, including the development of licensing examinations in nursing (http://www.ncsbn.org/regulation/boardsofnursing_boards_of_nursing_board.asp).

National Institute of Nursing Research

The National Institute of Nursing Research supports clinical and basic research to establish a scientific basis for the care of individuals across the life span—from management of patients during illness and recovery to the reduction of risks for disease and disability, the promotion of healthy lifestyles, promotion of quality of life in those with chronic illness, and care for individuals at the end of life. This research may also include families within a community context. According to its broad mandate, the institute seeks to understand and ease the symptoms of acute and chronic illness, to prevent or delay the onset of disease or disability or slow its progression, to find effective approaches to achieving and sustaining good health, and to improve the clinical settings in which care is provided. Nursing research involves clinical care in a variety of settings including the community and home in addition to more traditional health care sites (http://ninr.nih.gov/ninr/).

National League for Nursing

The National League for Nursing advances quality nursing education that prepares the nursing workforce to meet the needs of diverse populations in an ever-changing health care environment (http://www. nln.org/).

Nursing Organizations Alliance

The Nursing Organizations Alliance is a coalition of nursing organizations united to create a strong voice for nurses (http://www.nursing-alliance.org/).

State Boards of Nursing

Boards of nursing are state governmental agencies that are responsible for the regulation of nursing practice in each respective state. Boards of nursing are authorized to enforce the Nurse Practice Act and to develop administrative rules and regulations and other responsibilities per the Nurse Practice Act (http://www.ncsbn.org/regulation/boardsofnurs ing_boards_of_nursing_board.asp).

International Organizations

As consensus and action grow, a natural progression is to international organizations, of which the following three stand out.

World Health Organization

The World Health Organization (WHO) is the United Nation's specialized agency for the attainment of the highest possible level of health by all people. Its Web site (www.who.int) contains links to WHO projects, initiatives, activities, information products, and contacts, organized by health and development topics.

European Association of Palliative Care

The European Association of Palliative Care (EAPC) operates with the following aims:

- To promote the implementation of existing knowledge, train those who at any level are involved with the care of patients and fami-

lies affected by incurable and advanced disease, and promote study and research
- To bring together those who study and practice the disciplines involved in the care of patients and families affected by advanced disease (doctors, nurses, social workers, psychologists, and volunteers)
- To promote and sponsor publications or periodicals concerning palliative care
- To unify national palliative care organizations and establish an international network for the exchange of information and expertise
- To address the ethical problems associated with the care of terminally ill patients (http://www.eapcnet.org)

World Federation of Right to Die Societies

The World Federation of Right to Die Societies, founded in 1980, consists of 38 right-to-die organizations from 23 countries. The federation provides an international link for organizations working to secure or protect individuals' rights to self-determination at the end of their lives (www.worldrtd.net).

Lay Organizations

Lay organizations supply the grassroots interest and movement that can catch fire and put pressure on the health care system and the government to create *Golden Rooms*. A sampling of lay organizations is listed in the following.

American Association of Retired People

The American Association of Retired People (AARP) is a nonprofit, nonpartisan membership organization for people age 50 and over. This organization is dedicated to enhancing quality of life for all as they age. AARP endeavors to lead positive social change and deliver value to members through information, advocacy, and service (www.aarp.org).

American Cancer Society

The American Cancer Society is the nationwide, community-based, voluntary health organization dedicated to eliminating cancer as a major health problem by preventing cancer, saving lives, and diminishing suffering from cancer through research, education, advocacy, and service. The American Cancer Society's international mission concentrates on capacity building in developing cancer societies and on collaboration with other cancer-related organizations throughout the world in carrying out shared strategic directions (http://www.cancer.org/docroot/AA/content/AA_1_1_ACS_Mission_Statements.asp).

American Heart Association

"The American Heart Association (AHA) is a national voluntary health agency whose mission is building healthier lives, free of cardiovascular diseases and stroke. That single purpose drives all we do. The need for our work is beyond question (www.americanheart.org/)."

American Lung Association

The American Lung Association (ALA) has been a public health innovator for more than 100 years. Founded as the National Association for the Study and Prevention of Tuberculosis in 1904, we launched a nationwide effort to cure tuberculosis (TB) through education, research and advocacy, which became the model for today's public health programs. We created the first health education campaigns, sent health workers door to door, and advocated for laws to reduce the spread of TB, which was a radical departure from the charities and learned societies that existed at the time. By 1954, the death rate from TB was less than one-fiftieth of what it had been in 1904 thanks to effective public health policies and medications, developed in part through research funded by the association. In 1956, board members voted to expand the association's mission to include other respiratory diseases (http://www.lungusa.org/).

Alzheimer's Association

The Alzheimer's Association is the leading voluntary health organization in Alzheimer care, support, and research. Our mission is to eliminate Alzheimer's disease through the advancement of research, to provide and enhance care and support for all affected, and to reduce the risk of dementia through the promotion of brain health (http://www.alz.org/about_us_about_us_.asp).

Family Hospice and Palliative Care Association

This association provides support and care for people with life-limiting illness and their families (www.familyhospice.com).

Final Exit Network

This is the networking site for Final Exit members. Their goals are

1. To serve people who are suffering intolerably from an irreversible condition that has become more than they can bear
2. To foster research to find new peaceful and reliable ways to self-deliver
3. To promote the use of advance directives
4. To advocate for individuals when their advance directives are not being honored

Members believe that the needs of those who are suffering are paramount and applaud the work of organizations that seek legislative action to strengthen one's right to die a peaceful and painless death at the time and place of one's own choosing. They serve many whom other organizations may turn away. The Exit Guide program of Final Exit Network accepts members with cancer, amyotrophic lateral sclerosis (ALS; also known as Lou Gehrig's disease), Parkinson's disease, multiple sclerosis, muscular dystrophy, Alzheimer's disease, congestive heart failure, emphysema, and other incurable illnesses (www.finalexitnetwork.org).

SUMMARY

Engaging and building support begins with individuals taking small steps. Individuals coming together with small clusters of like-minded others can merge into organizations to build strategies for strength. Working through associations and organizations; using publications, media, and the Internet; and utilizing all the resources available can help carry us to our identified goals. Consider what you can do in your nursing or personal practice right now that will assist in honoring the life cycle and help move us collectively to better ways for peaceful, dignified deaths?

We continue to need resources to build on the support for dignified death at the end of life that is already present. We as individuals and organizations can express ourselves in voice and print through education, dialogue, the media, and politics. When we are united in mission, we can change the world.

WEB RESOURCES

http://www.aahpm.org
http://www.adec.org
http://www.worldrtd.net
http://www.hpna.org/
http://www.aacn.nche.edu/index.htm
http://www.who.int
http://www.eapcnet.org
http://www.aarp.org/
http://www.cancer.org/docroot/AA/content/AA_1_1_ACS_Mission_Statements.asp
http://www.americanheart.org/
http://www.lungusa.org/
http://www.alz.org/about_us_about_us_.asp
http://www.familyhospice.com
http://www.finalexitnetwork.org
http://www.congress.org/
http://www.compassionatefriends.org
http://www.aacn.org/WD/Practice/Docs/Designing_Agenda.pdf
http://www.aanet.org/
http://www.acnpweb.org/
http://www.ana.org/
http://www.aone.org/
http://www.ena.org/
http://www.ncsbn.org/regulation/boardsofnursing_boards_of_nursing_board.asp
http://ninr.nih.gov/ninr/
http://www.nln.org/
http://www.nursing-alliance.org/

REFERENCES

Carroll-Johnson, R. M. (2001). Nursing diagnoses at the end of life. *Nursing Diagnosis, 4.*

Chaves, E. H., de Barros, A. L., & Marini, M. (2010). Aging as a related factor of the nursing diagnosis impaired memory: Content validation. *International Journal of Nursing Terminologies and Classifications, 21*(1), 14–20.

Editor. (2007). *End of life: A nurse's guide to compassionate care.* Amber, PA: Lippincott Williams & Wilkins.

Klehr, J., Hafner, J., Spelz, L. M., Steen, S., & Weaver, K. (2009). Implementation of standardized nomenclature in the electronic medical record. *International Journal of Nursing Terminologies and Classifications, 20*(4), 169–180.

Müller-Staub, M. (2009). Evaluation of the implementation of nursing diagnoses, interventions, and outcomes. *International Journal of Nursing Terminologies and Classifications, 20*(1), 9–15.

Muller-Staub, M., Lavin, M. A., Needham, I., & van Achterberg, T. (2006). Nursing diagnoses, interventions and outcomes—Application and impact on nursing practice: Systematic review. *Journal of Advanced Nursing, 56*(5), 514–531.

"Nursing Care Plans End of Life/Hospice Care." Retrieved March 24, 2020, from http://nursingcareplan.blogspot.com/2007/02/ncp-end-of-life-hospice-care.html

Potter, P. & Frisch, N. (2009). Dying in peace. In B. M. Dossey & L. Keegan, *Holistic nursing: A handbook for practice* (5th ed., p. 146). Sudbury, MA: Jones and Bartlett.

Remen, R. N. (2006). Back to basics. *Kitchen table wisdom: Stories that heal* (2nd ed., pp. 44–45). New York: Penguin.

14 *Preparing for the Future*

Whatever you think you can do or believe you can do, begin it.
Action has magic, grace, and power in it.

—Goethe

*A*UNT LIL'S STORY   *Here's what I remember about Aunt Lil: She never forgot my birthday. Every year a card would arrive promptly on August 13. The colorful Christmas stockings she knitted for my brothers and me made holidays more magical. And when my dad got sick when I was 12, Aunt Lil was the one who told me he wasn't going to make it.*

Here's something else I remember, and it haunts me: When Aunt Lil had a debilitating stroke that confined her to a nursing home, I never once went to visit her. I can come up with all kinds of reasons—I was busy trying to find myself in New York City; she had a stepdaughter to take care of her; if she wanted to see me, she'd have asked. But the truth is, I don't recall that it ever crossed my mind that I should get on a plane and go to her. I can't fathom why, given how clearly I remember her pained words each time I'd call to ask how she was: "I'm just awful."

Then Aunt Lil died. Years later, when I asked my mom why we had let her suffer alone, she replied, "I don't like to think about it." I don't like to think about it either. (Graham, 2010, p. 4)

REFLECTIONS ON ISSUES OF CONCERN

1. How do you want to think about the end of life for your loved ones? Or don't you want to think about it either?
2. What does it mean to have a good death? Is this how others remember you? Is there more to it?
3. What are you prepared to take action on to change this type of thinking?

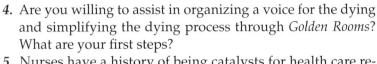

4. Are you willing to assist in organizing a voice for the dying and simplifying the dying process through *Golden Rooms*? What are your first steps?

5. Nurses have a history of being catalysts for health care reform. Where can you begin to speak and work for death with dignity?

6. "One small step for man; one giant step for mankind" were John Glenn's words when he landed on the moon. How can you network and work with others? What is holding you back?

7. At some point you will be dying. How have you prepared the way for yourself and others?

Shifting our consciousness to a larger perspective generally results in fresh ideas and new ways of seeing the present challenge. Within this larger perspective we begin to think outside the box of old ideas and ways of doing things. At first, the ideas might feel foreign, or we might think, "How can this ever happen?" With these thoughts it is best to keep an open mind and remind ourselves to follow our heart's desire of what is in our best interest for an easy and dignified death for ourselves and for others.

ORGANIZING A VOICE FOR THE DYING PERSON

As we learned in Chapter 5, "End-of-Life Costs of Care," the United States is spending billions of dollars on end-of-life care in acute care hospital settings and routine nursing home facilities. These costs are projected to increase exponentially as the baby boomers age and begin to die.

During the first decade of the 21st century worldwide, nursing health care professionals have accomplished and are at the forefront of health care change and accomplishments (Gennaro, 2010). Nurses continue to be the leaders in essential, emerging, and expanding health care areas (Hirschfield, 2009). Examples of some of these areas are seen in Table 14.1. Notice that in the emerging and expanding areas of health care, nurses are proactively embracing the changing clientele of the 21st century.

Also during this first decade health care costs not only rose but did so dramatically (Thorpe, 2005). Considering the escalating health care

TABLE 14.1   Examples of 21st-Century Worldwide Nursing
Leadership Areas

Health care essential areas	• Patient education
	• Preventative care
	• Symptom management
Heath care emerging area	• Palliative care
Health care expanding areas	• Long-term care
	• Gerontological care
	• Death with dignity/*Golden Rooms*

From "Accepting Responsibility for Long Term Care—a Paradox in Times of Global Nursing Shortage?" by M. Hirschfield, 2009, *Journal of Nursing Scholarship*, 41, pp. 104–111.

cost, it is vital to consider cost-effective ways to supply quality care. As is also apparent, the majority of Americans die in the hospital with numerous tubes, monitors, and invasive treatments. Our inner soul is growing in awareness, crying for the humane and gentle dignity of a death surrounded by family and loved ones. It is evident that the majority of those dying have no voice in this process. It is time for us as a nation based on religious freedom, liberty, and justice for all to come together and become this voice. It is time for nurses once again to be proactive within the health care system and be the change agent.

A GOOD DEATH

Just exactly what is a good death? And how does one achieve such a death? A good death has been described and gently referred to all through this book as one that has goodness, compassion, peace, dignity, and release. A good death begins when people come to grips with their own mortality and their own death and plan for their death both with physical preparation and by talking with family and friends about the end of life. As the dying and their families do their part, the health care providers also must do their part. A good death begins within the health care providers' self-care and personal inner work, which are needed before they can assist others. They also must become comfortable with their own eventual death. A good death means that the health care providers address and expand what is already the norm for most at the

Words of Wisdom

"**D**eath is simply the shifting from the form to the formless as expanding consciousness."

Drick (personal communication, May 17, 2010).

end of life and begin to change the norm. In effect it is time to raise the bar. In the final analysis a good death means that the family and health care professionals have a memory of a loving, peaceful, gentle death for their loved one or their patient. This is the time; here is the place for the *Golden Room*.

GOLDEN ROOM CENTERS

Golden Room centers appear to be the creation of the future, but in reality they are actually needed now. They are the next step in the palliative, hospice, holistic, shifting consciousness. By envisioning them we further set our intention to their physical reality. The question is always, "What is the next thing we need to do?" The present answer lies in developing individual *Golden Rooms* within already-existing institutions and building the first freestanding *Golden Room* centers. The grassroots support is already well underway.

Because Oregon and Washington led the way in the United States in end-of-life legislation and reform, it would be best if prototypes were developed here. These prototypes will set the bar for quality, care, and compassion as well as environmental aesthetics, support personnel and their preparation, and alternative modalities. Based on these prototypes additional regional centers can be established across the United States. Specific guidelines for the physical centers as well as the education of the personnel will be developed as the consciousness and demand to manifest these centers increase. A national certification for personnel working in *Golden Rooms* will be required.

Advantages of *Golden Room* Centers

The natural progression of any idea being set forth into reality is from a small to a larger conception until the reality takes on a life of its own.

In *Golden Rooms* this can be envisioned as individual clusters of rooms in acute care and nursing home settings, eventually evolving into free-standing centers. Freestanding centers present in themselves a unique set of advantages.

First, in being dedicated to the imminent end of life, they have no distractions in the form of other types of palliative care, as there are no survivors. As such, they become meccas for the most advanced and creative forms of physical atmosphere and creative comfort measures for both the dying and their families. A chapel would be available and nearby on the premises. Consulting and prayer rooms would be accessible. A play area for children would be available, as would soothing gardens with benches for families.

Second, both families and the dying would feel an immense sense of relief knowing that the entire staff is specially trained and concerned only with them and their situation. Third, an increasing number of acute care settings and nursing homes including physicians would relish the freestanding *Golden Rooms*. They would no longer have to deal with increasing mortality statistics as the U.S. population continues to age in larger and larger numbers. Fourth, insurance companies would relish *Golden Rooms* as an inexpensive solution to rising costs. Fifth, the humanity of death with dignity would return, and within a generation of *Golden Room* users and their families these freestanding centers would be seen as necessary, with an attitude of "How did we ever manage without them?"

The Ripple Effect

Interestingly, as these centers proliferate, they will be welcomed by both acute care settings and nursing homes, as they will no longer have to be concerned about their mortality rates since they can transport the dying to these centers. Suddenly nursing homes can change from a "place to go to die" to a place of loving assistance and help for those who need extra care. Acute care centers become a place for acute care, and many patients do go home. Lifting this burden from the back of the patient, the patient's family, and the health care personnel results in a feeling of expansion rather the contraction and dread that are usually felt. These patients can be given care without the underlying feeling of "they're only going to die anyway." Health care personnel can once again concentrate on their area of specialty and go home after their shift with a greater feeling of accomplishment and satisfaction. Continuing the cycle, as *Golden Rooms* are welcomed the demand increases for them. A gentle death becomes not a luxury of the few but rather an honored rite of passage for the many.

Individual *Golden Room* centers will be developed specifically for their setting: acute care, nursing home, assisted living facility, and eventually freestanding centers. Guidelines for the centers are crafted on the basis of the regional centers. The smallest minicenter would be five units replete with all the amenities of a regional *Golden Room* and with a separate staff from the rest of the facility. This staff would not be able to be pulled to another service area, as staff serving here have specialty training in death and dying in addition to deepening conscious awareness.

Golden Room centers can be located in acute care settings, nursing homes, and/or assisted living facilities, for example, situated at the end of the corridor or on a separate wing of the nursing unit. Each room will be a suite with special color lighting controls and comfort facilities for both the dying person and members of his or her family. If there is no family, then the personnel assigned to this unit would be able to be both attentive and comfortable. Staffing will be such that the personnel, in addition to delivering the customary care, can sit and talk with the person; offer complementary therapies, such as touch therapies and favorite foods; and fill other personal requests of the dying individual. Because of opportunities for these additional comfort options for the staff, as well as the dying person, the *Golden Room* setting will be seen as a desirable work area for staff, and many will likely opt for this assignment.

A person ready for the *Golden Room* setting will be able to request his or her favorite color, scents, type of music, films or television programs, foods, relaxed clothing, and other comfort measures. Once the options have been chosen, *Golden Room* staff will then arrange the lighting (e.g., a blue preference or a golden choice) and all other requests from a selection of lights, music, and aromas built into each individual room. Staff will be far more attentive and available than is possible with the ratios currently utilized in the majority of inpatient settings today.

As the awareness of the value of the *Golden Room* arises, the ripple effect will be seen in the quality of personal caring toward the dying person before he or she arrives in the *Golden Room*. Dying persons and their families will be eager to experience this growing humane and long-overdue rite of passage.

Golden Rooms in Acute Care Settings

Concomitant with the development of *Golden Room* centers, acute care settings undoubtedly will see the benefits and decide to establish *Golden Rooms* within their specific settings. This will follow a model much like that for labor and delivery at the beginning of life. Staff do not rotate in and out of this specialty area, nor would they be able to rotate in and out of the *Golden Room.*

Word of the *Golden Room* will spread among the general population. Older people and their families will begin to ask their physicians which hospitals have a *Golden Room* unit or offer transfer to *Golden Room* centers. Hospitals will discover that *Golden Rooms* suites are as necessary as birth suites. They will see the market for death with dignity. The potential for how *Golden Room* suites can change hospitals' philosophies and consciousness is exponential. And the families will be so thankful and eager, yes, eager to experience a return to this natural, humane rite of passage. The renal dialysis or critical care nurse who is told at the beginning of her night shift by an eager patient, "I waited for you to come," will become a thing of the past. There is no more waiting for someone to assist in the transition of the dying person. The assistance will always there in the *Golden Room.*

Golden Rooms in Nursing Homes

Nursing homes' version of the *Golden Room* will be complete with staff, environmental aesthetics, and family support within *Golden Room* suites. Since two-thirds of nursing home patients do not have family in the area, the specially trained staff will accommodate those special needs. The permanent *Golden Room* staff will also receive extra comfort measures in terms of sitting time, extra food, and a comfortable, quiet environment, thereby creating a desirable working atmosphere. Within a short span of time, personnel will be clamoring to take the required courses to qualify for these special positions.

PAYING FOR THE *GOLDEN ROOM*

Currently payment for nursing home care comes from one of three sources: Medicare, Medicaid, or private pay. Medicare and Medicaid, both of which are government funded, are running out of money. Likewise, many people have fewer savings than in the past. Something has to give. In truth, *Golden Room* centers will cost far less than most end-of-life heroic care currently rendered in the hospital. Current technological interventions complete with cardiac monitors, blood pressure readings, IVs and pumps, and feeding tubes will be gone. End-of-life care is now almost prohibitively expensive. With the advent and use of *Golden Room* centers, there will be no more billing for all the incessant, invasive treatments of today. Care will be palliative, comfortable, and spiritual. There will be the initial costs of developing and erecting Golden Room centers. However, once the rooms are built and equipped, the primary costs will be staffing, and because the staff will be offering comfort measures instead of treatments and IVs, costs will be significantly lowered. Insurance carriers should welcome the advent of *Golden Room* centers, if not for their humane approach to dying, then certainly because of the decreased cost to the payer.

ENLIVENING THE GRASSROOTS MOVEMENT

Deep within there is a place that knows truth, closer than your breath, deeper than your cells. As we feel these inner promptings and urges, we need to pay attention, acknowledge them, and move into action. For anything to change, to improve, requires responding to this inner place of truth and knowing. So what can we do to move into action and transform this idea that has come into its age into reality? What can we do to build and develop *Golden Rooms*? Exhibit 14.1 is a partial listing to get you started on a personal level.

As with any venture, as you take the first steps, more become obvious. You have to take the first step. The first steps begin with you taking action for yourself in preparing for the end of life both from the legal perspective—a living will, power of attorney, estate planning, and so on—and from a consciousness perspective—becoming comfortable with your mortality, talking about the end of life with your family and friends.

Once you have taken care of yourself, then it is time to move into the local area and share your ideas and thoughts. Exhibit 14.2 offers some suggestions to get started. You will discover more as you work locally. As you begin to talk and act on a local level you will be amazed at the contacts that you make and the interest that is created. Be willing to speak to any group. Even offer to speak to local clubs and organizations.

Finally, the ever-widening circle of contacts will lead you to the state and national levels as the next step. Exhibit 14.3 provides a list of helpful places to start. This is an interesting level to work at as you begin to draw attention to an idea that speaks to an issue that is near and dear to everyone. One question remains: Are you going to be part of the challenge

EXHIBIT 14.1   Personal Action Steps to Bring *Golden Rooms* into Reality

- Live more and more of your life in the present moment.
- Sit and envision what you would like for your end-of-life care. Write it down.
- Go online and find out about advance directives in your state. Get the forms for yourself, your parents, and your loved ones. Fill them out and include your preference to be in a *Golden Room*.
- Begin to reduce the size of the elephant on the table. Have heartfelt talks with family and friends about death and dying. It's healthy! What are their preferences? What music would they like? Where would they like to be? Let your family know your preferences.
- Check our blog: www.GoldenRoom.BlogSpot.com

EXHIBIT 14.2   Local Action Steps to Bring *Golden Rooms* into Reality

- Recommend this book to your local monthly book club.
- Ask the library to carry this book, or donate this book to your local library.
- Buy this book for two or more nurses or friends, then sit and discuss it.
- Call or email your local newspaper or television station and tell them about this book and the need to let people know about *Golden Rooms* as a progressive end-of-life option.
- Do a presentation on the *Golden Room* at your local professional nursing association meeting, women's or men's organizations, Toastmasters, nonprofit meetings, and so on.
- Talk with your health care provider and insurance agents about *Golden Rooms*. Do an in-service or Continuing Education Unit presentation.
- Talk with your local hospitals about the importance and advantages of *Golden Rooms*.

EXHIBIT 14.3   State and Federal Action Steps to Bring *Golden Rooms* into Reality

- Check to see what the statutes for the end of life are in your state.
- Offer to speak at conferences hosted by regional and national nursing and other organizations.
- Call your state and federal senators and representatives and let them know about the *Golden Room.*
- Send your state and federal senators and representatives a copy of this book.

or part of the solution? Are you going to read and agree that something needs to be done and do nothing, thereby remaining in the challenge? Or are you ready to say, "Yes, at some point in time death will happen to me and everyone that I love. This is important for everyone. This needs to happen and I can take action." The choice is yours.

FINAL THOUGHTS

In the final analysis the solution seems clear and direct. Let us as nurses

- Assist every person who desires a physical death with dignity to die surrounded by family or, if alone, to die surrounded by loving, caring people
- Assist the family to love and share the last moment of life with a loved one, giving them a sense of completion and wholeness
- Assist the family to avoid being faced with huge health care bills after the fact
- Assist the insurance companies to avoid paying out huge sums of money for needless end-of-life care
- Assist the state and federal government with health care reform

The *Golden Room* has benefits far beyond those stated, and these will be discovered as action takes place and this becomes a reality.

We have covered many questions, yet many details and refinements remain: Are there additional admission or acceptance criteria to be eligible for the *Golden Room*? Who decides? Would *Golden Rooms* be covered by insurance? How would the present health care system interface with *Golden Rooms*? Would government monies be available to build or add on *Golden Rooms*? What are the specific training criteria to work in the *Golden Room*? Would this training involve certification by a nationally recognized organization? Would this credentialing create a new specialty? Certainly within the planning stages all these seminal questions and more will be answered and clarified as we begin to reconnect with the natural flow of life from birth to death.

Transforming end-of-life health care is in part an internal evolutionary process. For one thing, nurses are evolving in valuing themselves. Creating and valuing ourselves and what we have to offer happens from the inside out. Each nurse can give birth to a genuine loving, caring, healing, spirit-filled practice that surrounds and enfolds all of humanity (Watson, 2006, 2008; Watson & Foster, 2003). This means going beyond routine nursing practice to assist in the transformation and awakening of the entire health care system. This shift in consciousness draws on the human spirit and visions of what might be—refusing to succumb to what is and no longer works (Watson, 2009).

One thing remains certain: It is time NOW to begin the shift to once again honor our elders, our children, our family, ourselves, and others by providing a physical death with goodness, compassion, peace, dignity, and release. It is time for the *Golden Room*.

Words of Wisdom

"Nothing lasts forever, not even the sun."

From Tolle (2005).

REFERENCES

Gennaro, S. (2010). Looking backward and looking forward. *Journal of Nursing Scholarship, 41*(1), 1.

Graham, N. P. (2010, March–April). Editorial. *AARP The Magazine*, p. 4.

Hirschfield, M. (2009). Accepting responsibility for long term care—A paradox in times of global nursing shortage? *Journal of Nursing Scholarship, 41*, 104–111.

Thorpe, K. (2005). The rise of health care spending and what to do about it. *Health Affairs, 24*, 1436–1445.

Tolle, E. (2005). *A new earth: Awakening to your life's purpose.* New York: Dutton.

Watson, J. (2006). Caring theory as ethical guide to administrative and clinical practices. *Nursing Administrative Quarterly, 30*(1), 48–55.

Watson, J. (2008). *Nursing: The philosophy and science of caring* (Rev. ed.). Boulder: University Press of Colorado.

Watson, J. (2009). Caring science and human caring theory: Transforming personal and professional practices in nursing and health care. *Journal of Health and Human Services Administration, 31*(4), 466–482.

Watson, J., & Foster, R. (2003). The attending nurse caring model: Integrating theory, evidence and advanced caring healing therapeutics for transforming professional practice. *Journal of Clinical Nursing, 12*(3), 360–365.

Index